Understanding Histamine Intolerance
&
Mast Cell Activation

By Mariska de Wild-Scholten

2013

3rd revised edition

COLOFON

ISBN:	978-1481283663 (printed)
ISBN:	978-90-818991-2-3 (pdf)
Title:	Understanding Histamine Intolerance & Mast Cell Activation
Author:	M.J. (Mariska) de Wild-Scholten
Publication date:	2013 March (third revised edition)
	2012 August (second revised edition)
	2012 April (first edition)
Publisher:	CreateSpace (printed)
	SmartGreenScans (pdf)
Keywords:	histamine intolerance, food intolerance, mast cell activation, mastocytosis, hypotension, migraine, irritable bowel syndrome, insomnia
Description:	Histamine intolerance and Mast Cell Activation result in allergy-like symptoms. Histamine-rich food or mast cell degranulators may cause diarrhea or constipation, low or high blood pressure, eczema, asthma, acid reflux, migraine, depression, rapid heart beats and breathing, panic attacks and sleep disturbances. This book describes the symptoms, assists in diagnosis and treatment. Basic knowledge is given to help patients to understand their enemy. Lists are included with concentrations of biogenic amines, mast cell degranulators and medicines which must be avoided. References and abstracts to scientific literature are provided as well.
BISAC category:	Health & Fitness / Allergies

Disclaimer

The information in this book is provided to the best knowledge of the author. The reader should consult a health professional before taking health related actions.

Please send comments to: info@histamine-intolerance.info.

Table of Contents

List of tables

List of figures

1. INTRODUCTION

Histamine may provoke direct symptoms like asthma, eczema, acid reflux, diarrhea and low blood pressure. There is a sensitivity to develop low oxygen levels in the blood which could give complaints like shortness of breath, cold feet, hair loss, muscle cramps, tension-type headache, depression, loss of short-term-memory. The body will try to increase oxygen input by increasing the heart- and breathing rate through the production of adrenaline. Excess of adrenaline may give migraine, anxiety, panick attacks, sweating, constipation, high blood pressure, sleep disturbances (waking up too early, nightmares). Women complain about painful menses.

Well known causes of high levels of histamine are infections and allergic reactions resulting in mast cell degranulation. What many people are not aware of (including health professionals) is that also certain foods contain histamine or degranulate mast cells. There are enzymes that degrade histamine but there may be a lack of capacity or activity of these enzymes resulting in high histamine levels. Some people suffer from instable mast cells and degranulation can be triggers by food components, fragrances and physical triggers like heat, cold, friction (itch from coarse wool) and exercise. Mast cells not only contain histamine but also other mediators.

Chapter 2 describes the stories of a few patients. It shows the often difficult path they took before they understood the root cause of the symptoms after which they could implement change.

Chapter 3 helps to understand what histamine and biogenic amines are, why they are present in certain foods and explains the fate in the human body.

Chapter 4 discusses the diseases resulting from high levels of histamine and mast cell degranulation.

Chapter 5 describes the possible cascade of symptoms. An attempt is made to organize the huge amount of complaints which could occur.

Chapter 6 discusses a few of the symptoms in more detail.

Chapter 7 assists in diagnosis, which is not easy because of a lack of acceptance and knowledge by health professionals.

Chapter 8 describes the different possibilities for treatment of histamine intolerance and mast cell activation including diet, medicines and enzymes.

Chapter 9 deals with treatment of hypoxia which may or may not be present as well.

Chapter 10 deals with treatment of dysmenorrhoea.

Chapter 11 shows the App "Histamine Intolerance" which includes most of the medicine and food list from this book.

Chapter 12 gives suggestions for scientific research. Many open questions still exist!

The **Appendix** gives tables of medicines which are better to avoid, food lists with histamine, other biogenic amines, inhibitors of enzymes, mast cell degranulators, salicylates, foods with lectin activity etc.

At the end of this book, **References** to books and articles are listed.

1.1. MOTIVATION TO WRITE THIS BOOK

From my own experience I know that it can take many years to find out the root cause of health symptoms. Health professionals see patients coming back again and again because their symptoms persevere. High costs are involved for medicines to treat the symptoms without knowing the cause, for ambulances and electrocardiography because a heart attack is suspected and for loss of working days.

The aim of this book is to provide practical knowledge and show to connection between all the symptoms to patients, health professionals, researchers and politicians and to increase the general awareness of histamine intolerance and mast cell activation.

For patients...

In the first place this book is written for patients. It is a practical fast and easy step-by-step guide for diagnosis and treatment.

The patient's only goal is to get rid of her / his symptoms.

Existing food lists often do not provide the reason why certain food items are on the list. This book aims at providing a better understanding.

For health professionals...

Histamine intolerance and mast cell activation is often overlooked. A quicker diagnosis is needed.

GPs (general practitioners) are the first health professionals consulted by patients so it is highly desirable that they have a general understanding of histamine intolerance and mast cell activation.

Dieticians can help the patients with the elimination diet and do the interpretation of the patient's diary. Good food lists are prerequisites.

Allergists are familiar with allergy and mastocytosis. However the leaking of histamine and other mediators from a *normal* (!) amount of mast cells is possible and must be recognized as well.

For researchers...

The fact that histamine intolerance and mast cell activation with *normal* amount of mast cells is not widely accepted by the scientific community does not mean it does not exist!

The abstracts of scientific literature are provided for reference.

For politicians...

A quick diagnosis of histamine intolerance and mast cell activation not only stops the suffering for patients, it also saves a lot of money!

There is a clear need for labeling the food with the histamine content at the moment of packaging. More funds are needed for research.

1.2. STEP-BY-STEP APPROACH: CURER

CURER is the fast and easy step-by-step approach to get rid of symptoms caused by histamine intolerance and/or mast cell activation:

Step 1: **C**heck if you recognize the symptoms of histamine intolerance and/or mast cell activation (Figure 2). Yes, then go to step 2.

Step 2: **U**nderstand histamine intolerance and/or mast cell activation. Read, read, and read.

Step 3: **R**egister in a diary what you eat, which medicines you take, other possible triggers and the symptoms you experience.

Step 4: **E**liminate the suspicious food and other triggers.

Step 5: **R**e-introduce the food/trigger after a while, in order to find out, if this particular food/trigger does or does not provoke adverse reactions.

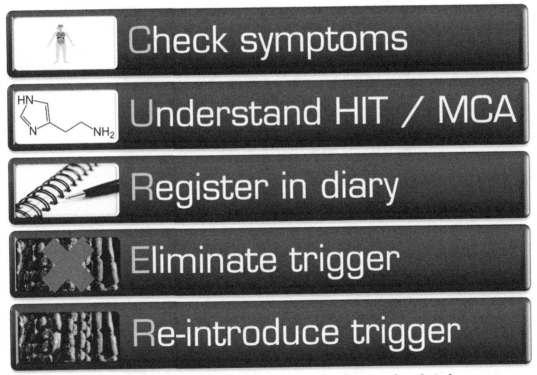

Figure 1 The CURER step-by-step approach to histamine intolerance and/or mast cell activation

Figure 2 Histamine Intolerance and Mast Cell Activation cascade of symptoms

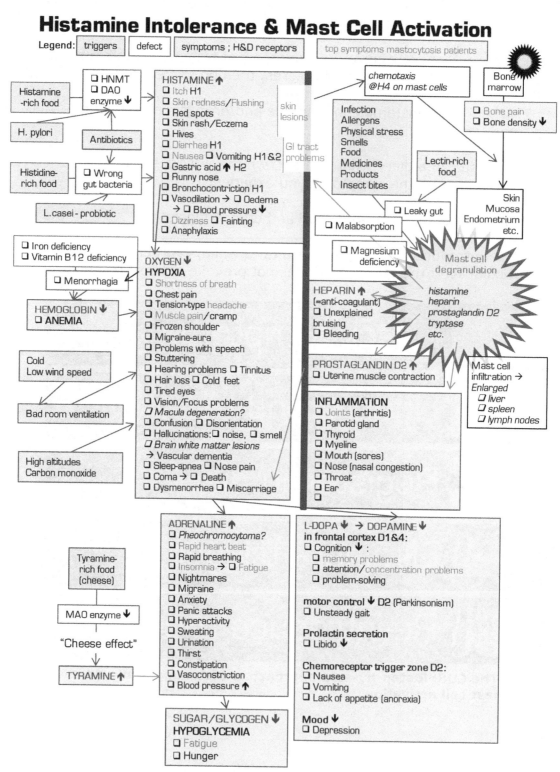

© Mariska de Wild-Scholten, www.histamine-intolerance.info, 25 February 2013

2. CASE HISTORIES

2.1. WOMAN, AGE 48, THE NETHERLANDS – THE AUTHOR

My monthly periods were always very painful (**dysmenorrhoea**) and this was associated with **fainting**. At the age of 19, on doctor's advice, I started taking birth control "pill" to get rid of these period complaints.

At the age of 30 **arthritis**-type of complaints started with a lot of back pain. Rheumatologists could not find the underlying cause. Erythrocyte sedimentation rate (ESR) was normal so it was concluded that there was no inflammation. Because of the stiff spine I was thinking it could be ankylosing spondylitis but X-ray images of the sacroiliac joint and the spine were normal and no HLA-B27 (Human Leukocyte Antigen B27) was detected in the blood. Later, because of painful cartilage of the ear after sleeping, I was thinking it could be relapsing polychondritis but the medical specialist did not want to investigate because the ear was never very red.
To summarize, there was no reason to suspect something "serious".
However I was unable to continue my job.
The day after my first and last visit to a sauna the pain was much worse.

At age of 31 I had an episode of **altitude sickness** when arriving at Toubkal Refuge (Maroc) at a height of 3207 meter. Headache, diarrhea, vomiting, even unable to drink water. Fellow travelers had no or limited complaints whereas I had to descent in the middle of the night.

After a few years the arthritis was replaced by chronic **headaches** (bilaterial, no aura, worse when moving around).

Around age 36 I had short episodes of **racing heart/irregular heartbeats**. At other moments I had **bowel cramps** without knowing what the cause was.

At the age of 38, I stopped taking "the pill" because of **headaches** starting on the first day of the stop week. Since then I live on ibuprofen to get me through my period days. One day, after the Christmas week I was too late taking ibuprofen with heavy diarrhea as result.

Although my headaches decreased, they did not disappear after I stopped taking anti-conceptives. So I went to my GP because of the headache complaints and asked if the cause could be a high blood pressure. I had a **low blood pressure**.

At the age of 40 my office work was becoming more and more demanding. How to get rid of the chronic daily headache? I spent my Christmas holiday reading about headaches on the internet. I often came across anti-migraine diets. Although I did not consider myself to have migraine, but just a headache (bilaterial, no aura), I said to myself that I should give it a try! What is there to lose? The food I decided to skip for some time was salami/chorizo sausages which I took often for lunch and orange juice.

During the same period, I went to a neurologist, specialized in headaches. His conclusion was that I suffered from 10% migraine and 90% tension-type headache. His advice was to take nortrilen (nortriptyline) for the tension-type headache. Furthermore, he recommended yoga and biofeedback therapy.

Surprisingly, after two weeks of my simple elimination diet the headaches were gone! Instead I became hyperactive, trembling fingers and unable to sleep and when sleeping I had nightmares, but the complaints slowly disappeared the following days. Bingo! So, I did not take the nortrilen and did not do any yoga/biofeedback because the problem was solved! Also I had the impression that I had less **hair loss**.

Then I started reading, reading, and reading. I asked the Dutch food information organization "Voedingscentrum" for a table with concentration of histamine in food (which they provided some years ago) but I found out that they have terminated this because they consider histamine intolerance scientifically unproven. Finally I found food lists in the book "Eetwaar = eetbaar?" by Dr. Kamsteeg and also I could get a copy of the Dutch ALBA list (1996) via a dietician.

The best information was only available in German language. I felt kind of lucky that I learned German at school! The book "Histamin-Intoleranz. Histamin und Seekrankheit" by Reinhart Jarisch (2004) really improved my understanding of the subject.

I was looking for a quick & easy test for diagnosis. Therefore, at age 41, I did a histamine blood test called "histamine in whole blood" in Dutch for 86 euro via the Klinisch Ecologisch Allergie Centrum (KEAC) in Weert/the Netherlands. The blood was taken when I was on low-histamine diet and without having health complaints but KEAC said that if I would have histamine intolerance this would be revealed in this blood test. The test result was that my histamine level was 37 µg/liter which is in the normal range of 28-51 µg/liter. The Dutch anti-quack society "Nederlandse Vereniging Tegen de Kwakzalverij" considers the KEAC to be quack. How reliable is this test?

I started keeping a diary for about 2½ years. The headache starts about 22 hours after the intake of suspicious food meaning at about 4 p.m. Eating the same meal for two days often gave no symptoms the second day. About one to two days after a an attack I was often suffering from **sleep disturbances/hyperactivity**.

At the age of 42 I went to an allergist and asked if he could prove my suspected histamine intolerance. He had to think about it. He is still thinking...

I suspected to have hay-fever because of **running nose, sneezing, red eyes** and headache but the blood test for inhalation allergy was negative.

At age of 47 I changed job and now work from home instead from an office. Very soon after this move I developed a **frozen shoulder** and **muscle cramps** in my upper arm. These cramps seemed to grow after eating oranges and disappear after taking Allerfre (loratadine: a H1 histamine antagonist drug).

At age of 48 I had **hallucinations** several times.
The first one was in Beijing, in a badly ventilated room, the day before start of my period. Early in the morning I heared people in the corridor making terrible noise. Also there was a disgusting smell. I had to throw up and had diarrhea. First I thought it was the food but when the vomiting did not stop I had the luminous idea it could be the start of the menstrual cycle and took ibuprofen which stopped the suffering. The next day I considered it impossible that there has been such a terrible noise and disgusting smell. I thought it must have been a hallucination, but since I was half asleep I was not completely sure. The next day, exhausted, I had my flight back to Amsterdam.
Next time, at home, at night, I heard terrible noisy people outside our house which did not wake up my husband. Later I thought this could have been another hallucination.
Another incidence, when arriving in a hotel room (windows closed), I heard terrible noise from a vending machine in the corridor. Next day I could verify this noise was non-existing. It was the day before start of menstrual cycle.
One night I heard in the forest next to our house a sound like someone was hitting a metal bar.
My last hallucination was at the moment of waking up I felt a kind of small metal ball falling onto my body. I immediately recognized it as being a hallucination.

Other complains around that time were: **shortness of breath (dyspnea), pain in top of nose, sadness, emotional crying spells, short-term memory loss, difficulty understanding fast speech, balance problems when walking, very tired eyes, hair loss, very very cold feet, tiredness, waking up very early with rapid heart beat (tachycardia) and rapid breathing (tachypnea)**. Symptoms were worse from ovulation to *end* of my period. I read about premenstrual dysphoric disorder (PMDD) but this seems to end when menses start. Menopause is starting?
Then, from Stans van der Poel I received tools to measure continuously heart- and breathing rate and breathing volume and was interested how the values would be for someone with histamine intolerance. In her office breathing rate was normal. When she put me into stress certain values improved whereas for "normal" people values would become worse. At home I monitored during sleep and I was shocked when I look at the

resulting charts. It showed episodes of very high heart- and breathing rates and moments when I stopped breathing (apnea; later confirmed by my husband) (Figure 3, Figure 4). I concluded I had difficulty getting enough oxygen: **hypoxia**!

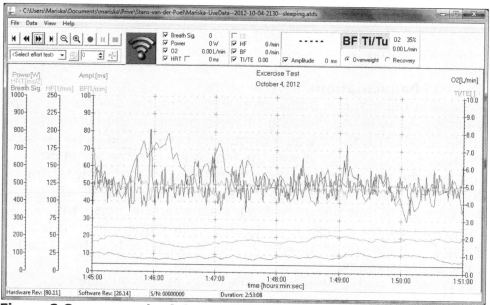

Figure 3 Somnograph of the author of this book

1:45-1.51 a.m. Recorded with a tool from Stans van der Poel: http://www.stansvanderpoel.nl/
Legend: Breath Sig = Breathing volume, HF = heart frequency (1/min), BF = breathing frequency (1/min).

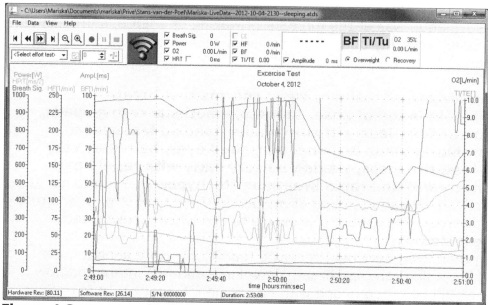

Figure 4 Somnograph of the author of this book
2:49-2:51 a.m.

My haemoglobin blood level was measured and in normal range (sample after end of period, in follicular phase of menstrual cycle).
I bought the Contec CMS50F finger pulse oximeter (110 euro) for continuous monitoring of blood oxygen saturation (SatO2) and heart beat (Figure 5, Figure 6). For different circumstances I can now check my oxygen saturation.

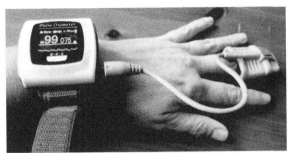

Figure 5 Pulse oximeter Contec CMS-50-F.

Blue: oxygen saturation (%), Green: pulse (beats/minute).

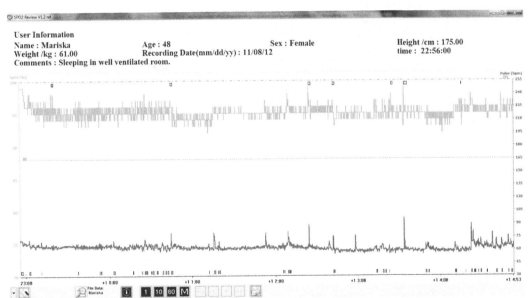

Figure 6 Pulse oximetry of sleeping in a well ventilated room.

Green: oxygen saturation (%), Blue: pulse (beats/minute)

In my office room at home there was no ventilation, except through the always-open door to the living room which has natural ventilation. But apparently that was not sufficient! From now on I tried to maximize fresh air 24 hours/day. It was absolutely amazing how fast my hypoxia symptoms disappeared. Only short-term-memory is improving very slowly. I take a one-hour walk every day.

A new natural ventilation grating (http://www.duco.eu/) was installed in the office room at home. Immediately I could measure an increased oxygen saturation when sitting in the living room and I can really feel the air flowing. Apparently you need two grating so the air can flow.

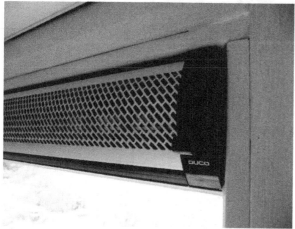

Figure 7 Duco natural ventilation system

A major defect was found in the **Histamine N-methyltransferase (HNMT) gene** (T105I) which codes for the enzyme Histamine N-methyltransferase resulting in a slower breakdown of histamine in the cells of my body (Figure 8). Bingo again! A saliva sample was analyzed by Novogenia GmbH (Mondsee, Austria) for 228 euro as part of their HNMT-study which investigates the relation between various defects in the HNMT-gene and histamine intolerance.

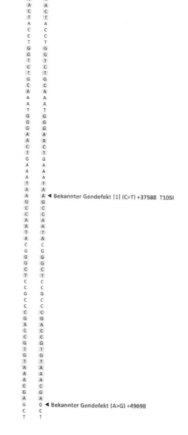

Figure 8 Histamine N-methyltransferase gene test results by Novogenia.

Yellow: important part of the gene, Grey: unimportant part of the gene.

Other symptoms:
- Terrible headache when I have a cold or flu.
- Don't like the smell of perfumes. Headache from flowering Cyclames plants. The smell of flowering Hyacinths is untolerable.
- Terrible headache a few days in February from something (fragrance?) in the outside air.
- After the first swigs of red wine I start coughing for a few seconds.
- Drowsiness after meals (somnolence). Caused by lack of oxygen for digestion?
- Eczema from contact with Rosin (Colophony). Rosin is a solid form of resin obtained from pines and some other plants, mostly conifers (Leylandii). The main component is Abietic acid. Rosin is used for example in plasters.
- Itching after contact with wool with course fibres.
- Eczema on elbows at pressure points, sometimes.
- Ice-cream headache (a short sharp headache after eating something very cold).
- Headache and tiredness from heat.
- Solar allergy: eczema from too much sun.

Suspicious food (*possible* culprits):
- Salami, fresh hering (histamine; nitrate vasodilator)
- Red beets, endive (nitrate → vasodilator)
- Wine-based vinegar like balsamico (acetaldehyde → mast cell degranulator)
- Raisins (sulphite → mast cell degranulator). Organic raisins without sulphite are tolerated.
- Citrus fruit (fragrances → mast cell degranulator)
- Spices in "ontbijtkoek", "speculaas", Glühwein (spices → mast cell degranulator)
- Green tea

Family member with HNMT-gene defect is intolerant to:
- contrast media (anaphylaxis),
- coarse wool (itch),
- formaldehyde and formaldehyde liberating in cosmetics (itch),
- tomatoes.

She uses the mast cell stabilizer Nalcrom when going out for dinner and there is no control over the ingredients.

2.2. MAN, AGE 55, GERMANY

Before he was affected by histamine intolerance himself, he knew the word "histamine" from a friend who told him, that in springtime (hay fever season) he avoided pork meat meals in order to lower his blood histamine level and thus decrease or even avoid the symptoms of his hay fever. Since he was affected by hay fever since the age of 19 too, he tried the same diet as his friend once, but without a convincing result. At an age of 50+ he encountered a couple of symptoms which could be avoided by low histamine food, as he learned later. For two years he was struggling with dizziness, "heart attacks", high pulse, constant coughing and red spots on his skin. He also experienced a couple of unclear collapses at the age of 53 which never could be traced back to a root cause. Electrocardiography (ECG) and Electroencephalography (EEG) showed normal results. Just as a test he was convinced by the author of this book to reduce or avoid some food which was considered most likely to contain high levels of histamine: canned fish, especially tuna and mackerel, salami, old mountain cheese. He got rid of the coughing within three days, and the beneficial effects on skin and heart slowly appeared. In the beginning of the test he experienced two nights without sleep and then felt much better than before.

For the supply of sausages he found a butcher using meat from local production without long transport distance for the animals and without industrial slaughtering. This reduces the stress for the animals and lowers the histamine level in their body accordingly.

Since this time his personal nutrition program consists of avoiding food having a strong negative effect, minimizing the food having unclear or weaker negative effects and concentrating on food having low or no effect as a basis for nutrition. Examples of these foods are given below.

By the way, his professional stress, has been at a high level since the age of 35, so there is no distinct difference in recent times which could explain an enhanced histamine level in his body. He ascribes his enhanced histamine level mainly to nutrition combined with the lowered efficiency of the diamine oxidase (DAO) enzyme because of his age.

Strong negative effect
- Gratinated cheese from convenience products, or in the restaurant, including (frozen) pizza dishes,
- Mozzarella,
- Smoked fish of any type, even fresh or high quality one,
- Canned fish, if more than 100 gram,
- Thai fish sauce,
- Cured ham, also as an ingredient in sausages or on sandwiches, one slice being sufficient for a negative effect, e.g. Wiener sausage or Bratwurst,
- Salami,
- Aceto balsamico of Italian type,

- Ice cream, UHT (Ultra-high temperature processing) milk or cream, also cream and tomato/cream sauces in restaurants,
- German Hefe-Weizenbier which is unfiltered white beer with yeast.

Weak negative effect
- Old mountain-type cheese, if more than 20 gram (there is a distinct difference between e.g. 6 months and 12 months old cheese from the same producer, the latter being more negative),
- Gratinated cheese homemade from freshly raped cheese, even Parmesan,
- White sheep cheese (greek type) if more than 100 gram at once,
- Large fish dishes (mediterranean type plates) with more than 250 gram of fresh fish,
- German type sausages,
- White wine vinegar,
- Mustard.

Low negative effect
- White cheese, fresh cheese especially from goat and sheep.
- Minced meat dishes, including burgers,
- Homemade lasagna,
- Dried mushrooms,
- Bread,
- Tomatoes, dried tomatoes,
- Homemade pasta Bolognese sauce,
- Potatoes,
- Chocolate.

No negative effect
- One glass (200 ml) of fresh milk has no effect, so there is no lactose intolerance.
- Salad and vegetables (including spinach) have no adverse effects.

Deviations from this diet have sudden effects, like strong coughing and/or diarrhea, three to five hours after ingestion. In addition, sometimes symptoms appear with a longer delay (heart, skin). So it is important to stick to the diet even after not recognizing an immediate effect.

At first, his general practisioner, taking care of his health since the age of 40, did not recognize this histamine intolerance when searching for the root cause for his dizziness and breakdowns at the age of 53. Remarkably, after telling that he had less symptoms with a low histamine diet, the GP commented that it appears "more often than expected" in his practice.

At age 55 a major defect (T105I) was found in the **Histamine N-methyltransferase (HNMT) gene** (Novogenia).

2.3. WOMAN, AGE 57, THE NETHERLANDS

Since her childhood she had very often metabolic disorders, related to food. She was fainting easily and had a low blood-pressure, all her life, up till the present day. Since the age of 29 she has **ulcerative colitis**. Since the age of 48 she has atrial fibrillation. At the age of 55 she was very ill, for over one year after a lung infection with asthma complaints.
She discovered the relation between histamine and her health complaints. Because of the ulcerative colitis she had already stopped with alcohol, caffeine, meat and fish, during the last 20 years. Also, since many years, she often has an acid reflux stomach.
Now she follows a histamine-low diet, which reliefs the abdominal pains and decreases the atrial fibrillation too.
Sometimes, she is tired and she still has a low blood pressure. In addition, she also suffers from rheumatism during the last 10 years.
Regrettably, a lot of physicians and nutritionists are unfamiliar with the histamine intolerance problems.

No defect HNMT-gene.

2.4. MAN AGE 52, FRANCE

At age 51 (January, 2011), he began having some odd symptoms. He went out walking one day, and felt his hands and feet **swelling** a bit; not seriously, but enough to bother him. That evening, at home, he felt a more generalized swelling all over his body, along with **flushing**. He took an allergy pill and, while it helped a bit, it didn't stop the symptoms entirely.
The next morning, he went to his GP who assumed that he had an allergic reaction to something. He gave him some cortisone pills to take for a few days, and his symptoms went away. But this occurred two more times in the following months, until one day he had a full-blown **asthma** attack. He had never had asthma before this, so I was quite surprised and scared. A couple of months later he got to the point where he was taking allergy pills daily, and he would get these flare-ups which didn't seem to correlate with eating any specific food or being exposed to specific plants. The internist in the hospital couldn't find anything, so he just went on taking his allergy pills and suffering from this odd swelling.
There was clearly something allergic going on. When someone would cut grass near his home, a village in the French Alps, surrounded by fields, he would swell up, and occasionally have trouble breathing. He was diagnosed as having allergic allergy and bronchial hyper-reactivity, and given an inhaler in case of problems. But all the allergy tests he had were negative, including those to grasses and standard pollens. He would often have reactions after meals - a half-hour to an hour after eating - and he started keeping a food diary, but was unable to find the food that bothered him.

At age 52 (January 2012), he moved to a large town an hour from where he had been living. He had hoped that some of his problems would subside being out of the country, but that wasn't the case. In addition to the problems that seemed related to allergies, he started having what he learned, from a gastroenterologist, was **irritable bowel syndrome**. He also suddenly became allergic to tomatoes, strawberries and red peppers; they **irritated his mouth, nose and eyes**. And red wine or sparkling wine would almost always lead to symptoms. He saw an allergy doctor in his new town who admitted that all this was beyond him, and he referred me to an allergy doctor at the hospital in Grenoble. Prior to this visit, he had the feelings that the doctors didn't take him seriously. He didn't have the usual allergy symptoms - massive edema (swelling) or **rashes**, but the doctor he saw seemed to immediately understand his problem. She asked him a number of questions about whether he was bothered by smells and perfumes (yes), whether he had a family history of allergies (yes, his mother), and scratched my arm with a pen. She then said that it was likely that he had histamine intolerance, and went on to explain a bit about it, and the elements that suggested this. Other than his physical symptoms, she said that people with pale skin (like him) were more likely to have it, and that they have rapid dermatographism (swelling on the skin where she scratched me with the pen). As for the tomatoes, strawberries and red peppers, she explained that these are mast cell degranulators and that, when he ate them, the histamine liberated in my mouth attacked my mucous membranes. She asked which meds he takes, and for most of them, just noted them, but when he said he is taking **diazepam (Valium)**, she said, "You take Valium?" with a tone of surprise. He does not take it often, mainly for the **dizziness caused by cavernous angioma in his brainstem** near the vestibular nerve, which was diagnosed in 2005, with symptoms from around 1982. He gets dizzy when walking more than about ten minutes and only takes small doses, 1 or 2 mg, because he is very sensitive to many drugs. He can't take more without getting sleepy.But Valium has a very long half-life, and that may have a long term effect. Also it's a DAO blocker, so he is going to try and find something else that can help with the dizziness. His neurologist had given him that both for the dizziness and the muscle spasms, saying that as long as he take it irregularly and in small doses, he's not worried about long-term use. He does not take it daily; sometimes every other day or so, sometimes a few times a week, depending on how he feels.

He has had many of the symptoms that are common to histamine intolerance: **irritable bowl, bloating, acid reflux, hypertension** (taking rilmenidine and lercanidipine**), dizziness, often after eating, coughing and asthma, flushing and arthritis**. At times, after meals, he gets very strong reactions where he had a **headache, dizziness, palpitations and tremor**. He'd also long had serious **muscle spasms in his back and torso**, which he attributed to a compressed nerve. A few years ago, they led to a painful **capsulitis (frozen shoulder)**. Interestingly, since he started taking antihistamines, these spasms have gone away. He has **arthritis** of the knees. The pain gets worse from time to time, but was pretty bad a few years ago. Since he has been taking antihistamines, it hasn't been too bad.

He is still in the testing stage, with a number of follow-up tests to be done very soon, so nothing is confirmed, but looking back at a food diary that he had been keeping for a year showed that the times when he had reactions after eating, there was at least one histamine-rich food in my meals. He ate a lot of fish, loved tomatoes, and often ate rice with soy sauce. But he had been looking for one single food that was causing his reactions; instead, it seems that dozens of foods were at cause.

Since then, he has managed to greatly reduce symptoms through changes in diet, eliminating all histamine-rich foods, and learning which foods cause symptoms. Avoiding fresh fish and meat, and only eating frozen, helps a great deal. A combination of two antihistamines daily, and low doses of prednisone when more acute symptoms appear, have turned this from a confusing situation into a minor annoyance.

2.5. MAN, UNITED KINGDOM

His symptoms were wheezing after drinking coffee, nausea, fatigue, disrupted sleep, loose and frequent bowel movements and hives.
He had been on a low histamine diet for 4 months, which was primarily poultry, vegetables and fats (also eating paleo diet). His health condition slowly worsened from day to day and things were getting pretty desperate. He also tried taking diamineoxidase (DAO) enzyme orally, which solved his gut symptoms, but did nothing for the other symptoms. Then he started working with a new dietary practitioner who asked him to do a stool sample which showed high levels of the bacteria **Helicobacter Pylori**. He started taking mastic gum to kill the bacteria at 1000 mg per day, just before bed, and after about 3 weeks he found himself able to eat beef again, and fish. His clarity of mind returned and his energy levels increased.
He was intrigued to find out why this might have happened, and after a little research discovered that H Pylori need vitamin B6 to thrive (Grubman 2010, Vitamin B6 is required for full motility and virulence in Helicobacter pylori, MBio. 2010 Aug 17;1(3), http://www.ncbi.nlm.nih.gov/pubmed/21151756). Vitamin B6 is also required to the production of DAO enzyme, which the body uses to break down histamine. So he guessed that the H Pylori had been using up his supplies of B6, making it impossible for his body to make enough DAO. This tied in with a test he had a year earlier, showing him to be deficient in vitamin B6.
So far his theory, but whether it is right or not, there is no doubt his histamine tolerance is much better than it was before. He may not be 'cured' yet, but his health situation has improved dramatically.
Supplementing Vitamin B6 may have worsened the H. Pylori infection!

3. UNDERSTANDING HISTAMINE

Histamine is a biogenic amine which means that it is an amine produced by natural biological processes. Other **biogenic amines** are for example phenylethylamine, tyramine, dopamine, noradrenaline, adrenaline, tryptamine, melatonin, serotonin, putrescine, cadaverine, spermidine and spermine (Table 1).

Table 1 Biogenic amines and metabolism

Precursor	Enzyme (process) Cofactor →	Name & Chemical formula	Enzyme (process) Cofactor →	Product	Enzyme (process) Cofactor →	Product	Enzyme (process) Cofactor →	Product
Histidine (amino acid)	L-histidine decarboxylase (Decarboxylation)	Histamine	HNMT (methylation) S-adenosyl-L-methionine = SAMe	N-methylhistamine	MAO-B (oxidation)	Methylimidazole acetaldehyde	Aldehyde dehydrogenase (oxidation) H_2O	Methylimidazole acetic acid
					DAO (oxidation)	Imidazole acetaldehyde	Aldehyde dehydrogenase	Imidazole-4-acetic acid
Phenylalanine (amino acid)	(Decarboxylation)	Phenylethylamine			MAO-B, MAO-A (oxidation) O_2	Phenyl acetaldehyde	Aldehyde dehydrogenase (oxidation) H_2O	Phenylacetic acid
Tyrosine (amino acid)	(Decarboxylation)	Tyramine			MAO-A+ (oxidation) O_2	Octopamine		
Tyrosine + O_2 → L-DOPA	(Decarboxylation)	Dopamine (a catecholamine)			MAO-A+, MAO-B (oxidation) O_2; COMT			
		Norepinephrine = Noradrenaline (a catecholamine)			MAO-A (oxidation) O_2; COMT			
		Epinephrine = Adrenaline (a catecholamine)			MAO-A (oxidation) O_2; COMT			
		Tryptamine			MAO-A, MAO-B (oxidation) O_2			
		Melatonin			MAO-A (oxidation) O_2			
Tryptophan (amino acid)	Tryptophan hydroxylase (TPH) & Amino acid decarboxylase (DDC)	Serotonin			MAO-A (oxidation) O_2			
Amino acids		Putrescine			DAO (oxidation) O_2	Spermidine		
Lysine (amino acid)	(Decarboxylation)	Cadaverine			DAO (oxidation) O_2			
		Spermidine			DAO (oxidation) O_2			
		Spermine			DAO (oxidation) O_2			

3.1. HISTAMINE IN FOOD

Histidine (an amino acid in proteins) can be converted to histamine by bacteria which is catalyzed by the enzyme L-histidine decarboxylase.

High storage temperature increase bacterial growth which results in high levels of histamine and other biogenic amines. Food rich in histidine (tuna) has the *potential* to generate high levels of histamine (Table 25).

In fermentation bacteria are added deliberately to give flavor to for example cheese, salami sausages, soy sauce or tempeh (Indonesian fermented soy beans).

Some types of bacteria ingested with our food (probiotics) or bacteria present in our gut are able to convert histidine to histamine (Table 2).

- Russo 2012: "*Wine <u>Lactobacillus brevis</u> IOEB 9809 can produce tyramine and putrescine under simulated human digestive tract conditions.*"
- Fernández de Palencia 2011: "*Here we report that tyramine-producing <u>Enterococcus durans</u> strain IPLA655 (from cheese) was able to produce tyramine under conditions simulating transit through the gastrointestinal tract.*"

Histamine is not destroyed during storage and cooking.
Histamine dissolves in water.
Histamine does not smell but other biogenic amines do. Trimethylamine has a fishy odor. Fresh fish does not smell!

3.2. MAST CELL DEGRANULATION

In the human body histamine supports our health system in the role of inflammatory mediator and neurotransmitter for example.
The granules of mast cells and basophils contain mediators like histamine, heparin, tryptase and prostaglandin-D2. An infection will degranulate these granules to liberarate/release the mediators which then attack invaders like bacteria, virussen, fungi and parasites.
Histamine may act as a regulator of mast cell degranulation (Carlos 2006).
Problems arise when not only an infection but also other harmless materials or stresses cause mast cell degranulation.
True allergy is the best known example. After contact with an allergen (always *proteins* like pollen) mast cells degranulate.
Other triggers may also degranulate mast cells which is then called sensitivity.

Table 2 Bacteria with decarboxylases which can convert histidine to histamine

	Bacteria with decarboxylases which can convert histidine to histamine:			Probiotic bacteria (in bold):					Bacteria in gut:	Fungi in the gut:
				Actimel	Danone Activia	Yakult	Brown Cow	Vifit		
A	Bacillus									
	Enterobacteriaceae									
A		Citrobacter								
A		Escherichia	E. coli						Escherichia	
A		Klebsiella								
A		Proteus								
		Salmonella								
		Shigella								
	Micrococcaceae									
		Kocuria								
		Micrococcus								
A		Staphylococcus								
A	Pseudomonas									
	Photobacterium									
A N	lactic acid bacteria (LAB)	Lactobacillus	L. acidophilus				**L. acidophilus**	**L. acidophilus**	**Lactobacillus**	
			L. arabinose							
			L. buchneri							
			L. bulgaricus	L. bulgaricus			L. bulgaricus			
			L. casei	**L. caseï Danone**		**L. casei Shirota**				
			L. helveticus							
								L. rhamnosus Gorbach & Goldin		
			L. sakei							
		Carnobacterium								
A		Enterococcus								
		Lactococcus								
		Leuconostoc								
		Pediococcus								
				Streptococcus thermophilus			Streptococcus thermophilus			
A N									Bacteroides	
A N				**Bifidobacterium animalis DN 173 010**			**Bifidus**		**Bifidobacterium**	

	Bacteria with decarboxylases which can convert histidine to histamine:			Probiotic bacteria (in bold):					Bacteria in gut:	Fungi in the gut:
								Bifidobact erium animalis DN 173 010 (trade name B. Lactis)		
A N									Clostridium	
									Eubacterium	
									Fusobacterium	
									Peptococcus	
									Peptostreptoco ccus	
									Ruminococcus	
										Aspergillus
										Candida
										Penicillium
										Saccharomyces
	Referen ces:									
	Koutsou manis 2010			http://en.wikipedia. org/wiki/Gut_flora	_	_	_		http://en.wikipedia.org/wiki/Gut flora	
	Legend:									
A :	Aeroob			**Bold: Probiotics in yoghurt**					**Bold: Probiotics in yoghurt**	
A N :	Anaeroob									

3.3. BIOGENIC AMINE DEGRADATION BY ENZYMES

Excess histamine and other biogenic amines are degraded by:
- histamine-N-methyltransferase (HNMT),
- diamine oxidase (DAO) and
- monoamine oxidase (MAO).

Table 1 shows an overview which biogenic amine is degraded by which enzyme. Biogenic amines compete with each other to be degraded. This means that biogenic amines may not cause the symptoms directly, but they can indirectly contribute to symptoms!

Because of the large size of the enzymes they are produced at the location where they are needed. The activity of the enzymes is different for each location in the body.

The enzymes can be inhibited by certain medicines (Table 13), biogenic amines and certain foods (Table 14).

Histamine N-methyltransferase (HNMT)

The HNMT enzyme catalyzes the reaction of histamine with a methyldonor to N-methylhistamine. The latter can be measured in urine samples.
The HNMT activity in different human tissue samples is given in Table 3.

Table 3 Histamine N-methyltransferase activity in human tissue samples

Human tissue	Sample size (n)	Mean ($\pm$ standard deviation) rate of histamine N-methylation in nmol min^{-1} mg^{-1} protein
Liver	60	1.78 $\pm$ 0.59
Kidney, renal cortex	8	1.15 $\pm$ 0.38
Kidney, renal medulla	8	0.79 $\pm$ 0.14
Intestinal mucosa	30	0.47 $\pm$ 0.18
Lung	20	0.35 $\pm$ 0.08
Brain	13	0.29 $\pm$ 0.14
Source: Pacifici 1992		

Diamine oxidase (DAO)

DAO co-factors are copper, vitamin B6 and vitamin C (Jarisch 2004).
Oral contraceptive use is associated with low vitamin B6 levels (Lussana 2003). Vitamin B6 is required for full motility and virulence in Helicobacter pylori (Grubman 2010).
DAO is continuously released from the intestinal mucosa.
During pregnancy there is a tremendous increase in the production of the enzyme DAO in the placenta to avoid miscarriages because the uterus is very sensitive to histamine (Szelag 2002, Maintz 2008). That is the reason why histamine intolerance symptoms disappear during pregnancy.

Aldehyde dehydrogenases

Aldehyde dehydrogenases are expressed at highest in liver, and at lower levels in many tissues (Crabb 2004). They oxidize aldehydes to carboxylic acids.

4. DISEASES

4.1. HISTAMINE FOOD POISONING

Eating fish with a high concentration of histamine can lead to histamine poisoning. Especially fish from the family scombroids (mackerels, tunas, and bonitos for example) are well-known for this; therefore it is also called scombroid poisoning.

There are legal limits to the concentration of histamine in fish food. Provocation test with exact legal-limit histamine doses resulted in mild symptoms and not in poisoning reactions. It is known that in cheese, for instance, much higher histamine levels are tolerated. Therefore, it is not correct to transfer the fish levels to other foods (Koutsoumanis 2010).

Legal concentration limits in fish and fish products: Europe

> STAGE WHERE THE CRITERION APPLIES: Products placed on the market during their shelf-life.
> - FOOD CATEGORY: Fishery products from fish species associated with a high amount of histidine.
>   UNSATISFACTORY IF:
>   - The mean value > 100 mg histamine/kg
>   - Or more than 2/9 values are between 100 and 200 mg histamine/kg
>   - Or one or more of the values > 200 mg histamine/kg
> - FOOD CATEGORY: Fishery products which have undergone enzyme maturation treatment in brine, manufactured from fish species associated with a high amount of histidine.
>   UNSATISFACTORY IF:
>   - The mean value > 200 mg histamine/kg
>   - Or more than 2/9 values are between 200 and 400 mg histamine/kg
>   - Or one or more of the values > 400 mg histamine/kg

Source: Commission Regulation (EC) No 2073/2005 of 15 November 2005 on microbiological criteria for foodstuff.

Legal concentration limits in fish and fish products: USA
Limit is 50 ppm (= 50 mg/kg).
Source: U.S. Food and Drug Administration, Fish and Fisheries Products Hazards and Controls Guidance, Chapter 7 Scombrotoxin (histamine) formation, (June 2001).

RASFF Food (Rapid Alert System for Food and Feed)
Histamine poisoning continues to be reported mostly in relation to tuna (RASFF Annual Report 2010).

Risk ranking

"The individual intake of the main food categories that contribute to histamine intake does not exceed the toxicological threshold of 50 mg. The food category being closest to the threshold is 'other fish and fish products' with an exhaustion of the threshold up to 83%. Consumption of 'fermented sausages', 'cheese', 'fish sauce' and 'fermented vegetables' leads to an exhaustion of the threshold of 74%, 64%, 60% and 55%, respectively. Nevertheless, the threshold may be exceeded by the intake of more than one food item containing high amounts of histamine during the same meal." See Table 26.
Source: EFSA 2011, p.56

4.2. HISTAMINE INTOLERANCE

Histamine intolerance is sometimes also referred to as histaminosis.

The recent German guideline (Reese 2012) summarizes important aspects of histamine intolerance and the consequences for diagnosis and treatment.

As described before, there are legal limits to the concentration of histamine in food, to avoid histamine poisoning. You can imagine that some people already get symptoms when the concentration is below this limit. This limit or threshold differs from person to person and may vary from day to day!
The underlying reason why some people are more susceptible is variable (Table 4). One of the reasons is a lack of activity of the enzymes DAO and/or HNMT which break down histamine in the body.

Because the symptoms are the same as with allergy, histamine intolerance is a pseudo-allergy, but it is NOT an allergy! Reactions occur with some delay and depend on the dose, meaning that it correlates with the amount consumed.

HNMT-enzyme
Defects in the HNMT-gene exist and certain polymorphisms results in a lower HNMT activity (Table 5).
Some medicines are known to inhibit the HNMT activity of which chloroquine is the strongest (Table 13).

Table 4 Overview of the multiple mechanisms of the Histamine Intolerance Syndrome (HIS) and a proposal for clinical classification.

HIS Group 1 (HIS-G1) through <u>increased availability of histamine</u> ("Histamine surplus" in the body)
- HIS-G1A: Endogenous and/or genetically intensified histamine synthesis and release
  - e.g: mast cell activation syndrome (mastocytosis), leukaemia etc.
  - e.g: atopy*, allergies*, infections, NSAID Intolerance
  - e.g: bacteria
- HIS-G1B: Exogenously raised histidine or histamine intake
  - e.g: food, wine, vinegar etc
  - e.g: blood products, tobacco smoke etc

HIS Group 2 (HIS-G2) through changes in the <u>histamine receptors</u>
- HIS-G2A: Genetically caused changes in sensitivity on the histamine receptors.
  - e.g.: genetic polymorphism (epigenetic changes?)
- HIS-G2B: Acquired changes in sensitivity on the histamine receptors
  - e.g: autoantibodies (?), infections, neurotransmitters, cytokines, etc.

HIS Group 3 (HIS-G3) through <u>impaired enzymatic histamine degradation</u>
- HIS-G3A: Endogenous and/or genetically caused enzymatic disorder at the level of Diamine oxidase (HIS-G3A-DAO) and/or Histamine N-Methyltransferase (HIS-G3A-HNMT)
  - e.g: genetic polymorphisms (epigenetic changes?)
  - e.g: bacterial amine production (constitutional, endogenous intestinal flora)
- HIS-G3B: Acquired enzymatic disorder at the level of Diamine oxidase (HIS-G3B-DAO) and/or of Histamine N-Methyltransferase (HIS-G3B-HNMT)
  - e.g: alcohol, medication etc.
  - e.g: ingesting biogenic amines (putrescine)
  - e.g: bacterial amine production (small bowel overgrowth syndrome (SBOG))

HIS Group 4 (HIS-G4) through <u>impaired cellular absorption</u> (?)

Source: Prof. Dr. med. Martin Raithel of the University Clinic of Erlangen (Germany), http://networkedblogs.com/EuTMW Masterman 2012)

Table 5 Defects in Histamine N-methyltransferase gene and association with diseases

(green: association, red: no association, purple: inverse association)

Polymorphism / Genotyping	Amino acid substitution	Alleles	Allele frequency	Associations / Functional and clinial impact	Sample group	Reference
	<u>Threonine</u>, <u>Isoleucine</u>					
C314T transition	Thr105Ile					Preuss 1998
		alleles encoding Thr105	0.900			Preuss 1998
		alleles encoding Ile105	0.100			Preuss 1998
A939G transition within the 3'-untranslated region		G alleles	0.790			Preuss 1998
			0.210			Preuss 1998

Polymorphism / Genotyping	Amino acid substitution	Alleles	Allele frequency	Associations / Functional and clinial impact	Sample group	Reference
				ALCOHOLISM		
	Thr105Ile	protective role of the Ile105 allele against alcoholism		Alcoholism: **inverse** association	German Caucasians 366 alcoholics + 200 controls	Reuter 2007
				ALZHEIMER		
	Thr105Ile	less active Ile105 variant	0.115	Alzheimer's disease	Croatian 256 AD	Marasovic 2011
			0.134	healthy controls	Croatian 1190 healthy controls	Marasovic 2011
				ASTHMA & ALLERGIC RHINITIS		
rs1801105 (314C/T)	Thr105Ile	TT genotype and T allele		Asthma	149 asthmatic children + 156 healthy children	Szczepankiewicz 2010
rs2071048 (-1637T/C)						Szczepankiewicz 2010
rs11569723 (-411C/T)						Szczepankiewicz 2010
rs1050891 (1097A/T)						Szczepankiewicz 2010
	Thr105Ile		0.160	Asthma	270 Asthma and/or allergic rhinitis + 295 healthy controls	Garcia-Martin 2007
			0.132	Allergic rhinitis		Garcia-Martin 2007
			0.115	Controls		Garcia-Martin 2007
C314T				Asthma: no association	Indian population	Sharma 2005
A929G						Sharma 2005
(CA)n repeat in intron 5						Sharma 2005
(CA)n repeat (BV677277)						Sharma 2005
				DUODENAL ULCER		
C314T		T314 allele	0.033	Duodenal ulcer: no association	Chinese 498 DU	Hailong 2008
		T314 allele	0.035		Chinese 151 healthy controls	Hailong 2008
		C/C genotypes	0.930		Chinese 498 DU	Hailong 2008
		C/C genotypes	0.934		Chinese 151 healthy controls	Hailong 2008

Polymorphism / Genotyping	Amino acid substitution	Alleles	Allele frequency	Associations / Functional and clinial impact	Sample group	Reference
		T/T genotype	not found			Hailong 2008
				ECZEMA		
C314T	Thr105Ile			Atopic dermatitis	249 Caucasian children	Kennedy 2008
314C>T				Eczema, non-atopic	763 Korean children	Lee 2012
413C>T				Eczema: no association		Lee 2012
465T>C				Eczema: no association		Lee 2012
939A>G				Eczema in the atopy groups		Lee 2012
				MIGRAINE		
C314T (on exon 4)	Thr105Ile			Migraine: no association		Garcia-Martin 2008
				MS		
	Thr105Ile			Multiple sclerosis: no association		Garcia-Martin 2010
				PARKINSON & ESSENTIAL TREMOR		
	Thr105Ile			Parkinson's disease	913 PD + 958 controls	Palada 2012
rs11558538	Thr105Ile	threonine allele		Parkinson's disease and Essential tremor: no association		Keeling 2010
	Thr105Ile	higher frequency of homozygous HNMT 105Thr genotypes leading to high metabolic activity		Essential tremor	204 ET + 295 healthy controls	Ledesma 2008
	Thr105Ile			Parkinson's disease	214 PD + 295 healthy controls	Agundez 2008
				ULCERATIVE COLITIS		
	Thr105Ile			Ulcerative colitis	229 UC + 261 controls	Garcia-Martin 2006
				URTICARIA		
314C>T				Urticaria, aspirin intolerant chronic: no association		Kim 2009
939A>G				Urticaria, aspirin intolerant chronic		Kim 2009
				VARIOUS		
	Thr105Ile			Parkinson's disease, essential tremor, attention-deficit hyperactivity disorder (ADHD), asthma and alcoholism		in: Marasovic 2011

DAO-enzyme
Some food and medicines may inhibit the function of the enzyme DAO.

Defects in the DAO-gene exist.
"Among all polymorphisms found in DAO sequence, it has been proved that only one of the 7 polymorphisms, (with reference rs1049793) located in the third exon, has relation with low DAO activity. Carriers of this polymorphism, present lower DAO activity than controls with significant effect. Preliminary studies suggest that this polymorphism has an overall prevalence close to 0.30 (30% of mutated alleles). Other studied polymorphisms of the same type of substitution of amino acids, do not show changes in enzyme DAO activity."
Citation from http://www.deficitdao.org/en/factores-geneticos.php#.UBTtCbT0h8E (28 July 2012).

Inflammatory Bowel Diseases (IBD) like Ulcerative Colitis and Crohn's disease have a decreased DAO activity in the bowel (Table 6).

Ulcerative Colitis (UC) is a chronic inflammation (*...itis*) of the colon (*Col....*) with generation of ulcers (*Ulcerative*). In UC patients a lower DAO activity was found. In UC patients where the UC was in remission a much higher DAO activity was found (Mennigen 1990).

Crohn's disease (regional enteritis) is a chronic inflammation of the gastrointestinal tract from mouth to anus. Diseased mucosa has significantly lower DAO activity.

Table 6 DAO activity in normal humans and in patients with Ulcerative Colitis or Crohn's disease

Patients & Controls	number of samples (n)	DAO activity in nmol/min g	Reference
ULCERATIVE COLITIS (UC)			
Normal	30	22.8	Mennigen 1990
UC	12	2.7	Mennigen 1990
UC in remissions	3	103, 107, 208	Mennigen 1990
CROHN'S DISEASE			
Crohn, normal gut, proximal		155.6 (76-393)	Schmidt 1990
Crohn, normal gut, distal		132 (58.5-295)	Schmidt 1990
Crohn, diseased gut		74.5 (5-262)	Schmidt 1990

MAO-enzyme
Some foods and medicines are known to inhibit the MAO-A and/or MAO-B enzymes (Table 14).

4.3. HISTADELIA/UNDERMETHYLATION QUACKERY

*"Histadelia" is a condition hypothesised by Carl Pfeiffer to involve elevated serum levels of histamine and basophils, which he says can be treated with methionine and vitamin B6 **mega**doses. Pfeiffer claims that "histadelia" can cause depression with or without psychosis, but no published clinical trials have tested the effectiveness of this therapy.*
Source: http://en.wikipedia.org/wiki/Orthomolecular_psychiatry#Histadelia

Histadelia / undermethylation is theory is part of orthomolecular medicine:
http://en.wikipedia.org/wiki/Orthomolecular_medicine

Methionine
One pathway for the degradation of histamine in the body is via the reaction of histamine with the methyldonor methionine to N-methylhistamine:

Histamine
+
S-Adenosyl-L-methionine

 *

N-Methylhistamine
+
S-Adenosyl-homocysteine

* This reaction is accelerated by the enzyme histamine N-methyltransferase (HNMT).

"Methionine is an essential amino acid meaning the human cannot synthesize it so you need to eat it. High levels of methionine can be found in eggs, sesame seeds, Brazil nuts, fish, meats and some other plant seeds. A 2009 study on rats showed "methionine supplementation in the diet specifically increases mitochondrial ROS production and mitochondrial DNA oxidative damage in rat liver mitochondria offering a plausible mechanism for its hepatotoxicity".
http://en.wikipedia.org/wiki/Methionine

Vitamin B6
Vitamin B6 is a cofactor for the enzyme diamine oxydase.
Good sources of vitamin B6 include meats, whole grain products, vegetables, nuts and bananas.
High doses of vitamin B6 can be toxic.
http://en.wikipedia.org/wiki/Vitamin_B6

Mental symptoms like depression
Histamine intolerance combined with low oxygen levels (for example from badly ventilated rooms) may cause hypoxia with mental (and other) problems as a result.

Conclusions:
- Avoid high levels of histamine.
- Optimize oxygen levels in your body.
- Supplements of methionine and vitamin B6 are not needed when you eat well balanced.
- *MEGA*doses of methionine and vitamin B6 may be toxic!

4.4.   TYRAMINE INTOLERANCE

Tyramine is metabolized by the MAO_A enzyme. Tyramine causes the release of adrenaline which results in high blood pressure. Medicines which inhibit the MAO enzyme (MAOI) therefore can lead to fatal high blood pressure when combined with high-tyramine food.

- *"The individual intake of the main food categories that contribute to tyramine intake does not exceed the toxicological threshold of <u>600 mg</u>. Even if the five main sources were combined at the same meal, their contribution would be of 77% of the 600 mg tyramine threshold.*
- *The high exposure values estimated for beer, cheese, fermented sausages and fermented meat fish substantially exceed (from 180.8 to 249.2%) the <u>50 mg</u> threshold for individuals taking reversible and selective (3rd generation) MAOI drugs.*
- *For highly sensitive consumers, i.e. those under classical MAOI medication, the estimated threshold level <u>6 mg</u> is easily reached by the consumption of fermented foods. Therefore, these sensitive individuals should avoid all tyramine containing food."*

Source: EFSA 2011, p. 56-57.

4.5. MAST CELL ACTIVATION

In sensitive people mast cells and basophils not only degranulate after an infection (bacteria, virus, fungi, parasite) but also by the following **triggers**:

1. Allergens (dust mite excretion, pollen),
2. Insect bites,
3. Physical stress (heat, cold, pressure, friction, exercise, solar light),
4. Chemicals in the air (perfumes, tobacco smoke, pollution),
5. Products (personal care, furniture),
6. Medicines,
7. Medical agents (contrast media),
8. Food additives (benzoate, sulfite etc.),
9. Food components (citral in citrus fruit peel etc.),
10. Food metabolites (acetaldehyde from alcohol).

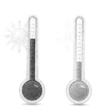

Allergy is a well-accepted cause of mast cell degranulation.
Allergic reactions are immediate and can occur after contact with only small traces of an allergen.
A true food allergy requires the presence of Immunoglobin E (IgE) antibodies against the food. Allergens are always *proteins*. Allergenic foods included in Annex IIIa of Directive 2000/13/EC, 2003/89/EC, 2007/68/EC (European Commission) are:

- Fish
- Crustaceans
- Molluscs
- Eggs
- Milk
- Cereals
- Peanuts
- Soybeans
- Nuts i.e. almonds (Amygdalus communis L.), hazelnuts (Corylus avellana), walnuts (Juglans regia), cashews (Anacardium occidentale), pecan nuts (Carya illinoiesis (Wangenh.) K. Koch), Brazil nuts (Bertholletia excelsa), pistachio nuts (Pistacia vera), macadamia nuts and Queensland nuts (Macadamia ternifolia)
- Mustard
- Sesame
- Celery
- Lupin

Non-allergic mast cell degranulation is also possible.
One food included in Annex IIIa of Directive 2000/13/EC, 2003/89/EC, 2007/68/EC (European Commission) is sulphur oxide/sulphites.
Established fragrance contact allergens are listed in the Appendix. Many of these components ("aroma", limonene, linalool, vanillin, menthol) can be

present in food (bay laurel, cinnamon, clove, citrus fruit peel, and peppermint). We can expect adverse effects when they are digested by sensitive people. Unfortunately oral challenge studies on established (fragrance) contact allergens are lacking. Blood tests are not avaible. More research in needed in this area!

Mastocytosis is a disease where the number of mast cells is increased. In **Mast Cell Activation Syndrome** the number of mast cells is normal but they degranulate easily (Hermine 2008, Hamilton 2011, Frieri 2012, Valent 2012).

4.6.   LEAKY GUT BY LECTINS & SALICYLATES

A leaky gut is intestinal hyperpermeability. Increased permeability of the gut can lead to increased sensitivities towards food ingredients.

✓ Low-lectin diet

Lectins are sugar-binding proteins. Every type of lectin binds to specific sugar structures and by this mechanism they can damage the gut epithelial cells. Lectins then enter the body and cause damage to for example cartilage tissue. Some lectins bind to N-acetyl glucosamine explaining the use of glucosamine-based supplement in the treatment of arthritis.
In addition the lectin phytohaemagglutinin (PHA) which is found in beans causes mast cell degranulation.
Table 29 indicates lectin activity in food. Especially legumes, grains and nightshades are high in lectin.

✓ Low-salicylate diet

Salicylates depress the production of protective glycoproteins.

4.7.   HELICOBACTER PYLORI INFECTION

Helicobacter pylori is a bacteria which may be present in the stomach. Vitamin B6 is required for full motility and virulence in Helicobacter pylori (Grubman 2010). Vitamin B6 is also required to the production of DAO enzyme, which the body uses to break down histamine!
Various studies showed the disappearance or reduction of migraine headache after eradication of the Helicobacter pylori infection (Gasbarrini 1998, Yiannopoulou 2007, Hosseinzadeh 2011, Faraji 2012).

5. CASCADES OF SYMPTOMS

In this chapter possible symptoms of histamine intolerance and mast cell degranulation are discussed. Usually, only a few of the symptoms are experienced. The symptoms could be a sign of a different disease.

It is extremely important to consider *all* symptoms because it helps to find the root cause and triggers. Finding the *not-always-so-obvious* triggers means we have the opportunity to avoid them and to stop taking expensive medicines which only treat symptoms and which may have unwanted side-effects.

The goal was to organize the symptoms and look for the connection. This modeling of the cascade of symptoms (Figure 2) is the interpretation of the author of this book and is based on own experience, reading of wiki-pages and literature. Direct primary symtoms of increased concentration of histamine may or may not be followed by indirect symptoms (hypoxia → adrenaline → hypoglycemia). Bronchoconstriction leads to the danger that you do not manage to get enough oxygen to the blood (hypoxia). Lack of oxygen triggers the body to increase breathing- and heart rate by increasing adrenaline concentration. A high heart beat means you will consume sugar & glucogen for fast energy supply instead of slow burning of fat. Sugar/glycogen supplies are very limited so you may end up with hypoglycemia (low blood sugar). It is not always easy to put a symptom in the right "box" because symptoms may take place almost simultaneously.

5.1. HISTAMINE

Histamine acts via histamine receptors (H1, H2, H3, H4) and causes symptoms in different parts of the body:
- SKIN@H1: itch (pruritis), hives (urticaria), rashes (eczema), flush, red skin,
- STOMACH @H2: stimulation of gastric acid secretion,
- INTESTINE/BOWEL/GUT @H1: ileum contraction, diarrhea, bowel cramp, irritable bowel,
- RESPIRATORY TRACT: runny nose, nasal congestion, sneezing, sore throat, cough, @H1 bronchoconstriction (asthma),
- EYES@H1: itch,
- BLOOD VESSELS @H1: vasodilation, low blood pressure (hypotension) and as a result leaking of fluids (oedema),
- MAST CELLS @H4: mediate mast cell chemotaxis which is the migration of mast cells.

"Histamine was shown to mediate signaling and chemotaxis of mast cells via the H4 receptor. This mechanism might be responsible for mast cell accumulation in allergic tissues."
Hofstra 2003.

"The human histamine H(4) receptor is mainly expressed in cells of the human immune system (e.g. mast cells, eosinophils, monocytes, dendritic cells, T cells) and mediates several effects on chemotaxis with numerous cell types."
Walter 2011

Is this the link why histamine intolerance patients often also have problems with their mast cells?

5.2. HYPOXIA: LOW OXYGEN

Hypoxia is defined as a deficiency of oxygen in the body (tissue).
Hypoxemia is defined as a deficiency of oxygen in arterial blood.

Hypoxia can be a secondary symptom of high histamine:
"A 25-year-old woman with documented mastocytosis developed hypoxemia with pruritus, diarrhea, headache, and hypotension on two separate occasions. The hypoxemia appeared to be related to a massive release of histamine. Resolution of the patient's symptoms was accompanied by the return of her arterial oxygen tension to normal levels." Kaye 1979.

Bronchoconstriction restricts the uptake of oxygen in the blood. This means there is a higher sensitivity to low oxygen levels (for example badly ventilated rooms and high altitudes) compared to "normal" people.

Table 7 shows an overview of possible symptoms from hypoxia experienced by for example patients who suffer from anemia, sleep apnea, altitude/mountain sickness or carbon monoxide poisoning. The body will respond by increasing heartbeat (tachycardia) and breathing rate (tachypnea) via the release of adrenaline. So some symptoms are from hypoxia and some are from adrenaline.

Lack of oxygen:
- Dizziness,
- Cold feet, loss of hair (the extremities),
- Muscle cramp, frozen shoulder?!,
- Tension-type headache,
- Auro before migraine,
- Tired eyes,
- Problems with vision (focusing),
- Macula degeneration?!
- Problems with speech,
- Confusion, Disorientation,
- Hallucinations (noise, smells),
- Tinnitus,
- Sleapiness (somnolence) especially after heavy meals.
- Brain white matter lesions,
- Coma,
- Death.

Dopamine is produced in the brain from levo-dopa:

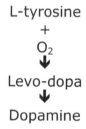

L-tyrosine
+
O_2
↓
Levo-dopa
↓
Dopamine

The production of levo-dopa requires oxygen (O_2)! Decreased levels of dopamine results in the following symptoms:
- Unsteady gait/walk,
- Loss of short-term memory,
- Nausea, vomiting,
- Lack of appetite,
- Sadness, depression,
- Decreased libido.

A depression from lack of dopamine will not respond to treatments to increase serotonine!

5.3. ADRENALINE

After anaphylaxis a fast injection with adrenaline is needed. The body can also produce adrenaline in the adrenal gland! When your body senses a lower oxygen saturation (below 95% SatO2?) it will increase the heart- and breathing rate (by increasing adrenaline) to increase the uptake of oxygen.

If one day you have symptoms from certain food and you eat the next day the same food you may not experience symptoms because your body has adapted. Also if the body has been on a high level of histamine for some time and the histamine concentration is suddenly decreased your adrenaline may still be too high resulting in sleepless nights etcetera.

Symptoms from adrenaline:
- Rapid heart beat,
- Rapid breathing,
- Insomnia resulting in tiredness,
- Nightmares,
- Migraine,
- Anxiety,
- Panic attacks,
- Hyperactivity,
- Sweating,
- Urination,
- Thirst,
- Constipation,
- Vasoconstriction,
- High blood pressure (hypertension).

Could you develop a pheochromocytoma (enlarged adrenal gland) after a life-long histamine intolerance?

Table 7 Symptoms of hypoxia

Sources: Wiki & http://www.anesthesiaweb.org/hypoxia.php

Symptoms of hypoxia		Hypoxia	Hypoxia	Hypoxia	Anemia	Sleep apnea	Altitude sickness	Altitude sickness	Chronic mountain sickness	Carbon monoxide poisoning	Carbon monoxide poisoning
		Moderate	Severe	Extreme			Primary	Severe		Acute	Chronic
	Oxygen saturation, SpO2:	80-60%	60-40%	<40%							
Respiratory:	Dyspnea (Shortness of breath)				x				x		
Respiratory:	Dyspnea (Shortness of breath) upon exertion				x		x	x			
Respiratory:	Abnormal breathing			x							
Nose:	Nosebleed						x	x			
Heart:	Palpitations (abnormality of heartbeat), cardiac arrhythmia				x				x	x	
Heart:	Tachycardia (fast heart rate), rapid pulse				x		x	x		x	
Heart:	Chest pain, angina, heart attack				severe						
Blood vessels:	Hypotension (low blood pressure)				x					x	
Blood vessels:	Dilation of veins								x		
Brain:	Headache						x	x	x	x	x
Brain:	Dizziness or lightheadedness				x		x	x	x	x	x
Brain:	Seizures, fainting				severe					x	
Brain:	Difficulty with higher intellectual functions									delayed	
Brain:	"executive functioning": planning and initiating tasks					x					
Brain:	Attention: difficulty in paying attention, working effectively and processing information					x					
Brain:	Attitude of serene unconcern, of calm and tranquil indifference to everything, including pain, or even hilarity, euphoria, to a sense of power with ultimate knowledge.	x									
Brain:	Decreased attentiveness and drive					x					
Brain:	Reduced ability to remember and recognize	x									
Brain:	Amnesia (memory loss)					x				delayed	x
Brain:	Short-term memory loss					x				delayed	

Symptoms of hypoxia		Hypoxia	Hypoxia	Hypoxia	Anemia	Sleep apnea	Altitude sickness	Altitude sickness	Chronic mountain sickness	Carbon monoxide poisoning	Carbon monoxide poisoning
Brain:	Reduced ability to perform word association tests, together with causing abnormal responses	x									
Brain:	Unable to speak, speech disturbances		x							delayed	
Brain:	Slower reaction times	x									
Brain:	Slower speech comprehension	x									
Brain:	Reduced performance in intelligence tests	x									
Brain:	Reduced hand steadiness, and degrades visual contrast discrimination	x									
Brain:	Feelings of "sensed presence" - a sensation where the affected person senses the presence of a person or other being in their vicinity	x									
Brain:	Feelings of depersonalization, and van even induce out-of-body experiences	x									
Brain:	Moodiness					x					
Brain:	Depression									x, delayed	x
Brain:	Belligerence (acting in a hostile manner)					x					
Brain:	Conscious but paralyzed, and cannot move, even when they try		x								
Brain:	Immobility of the eyes, which then stare straight ahead		x								
Brain:	Irritability									delayed	
Brain:	Delirium									x	
Brain:	Psychosis									delayed	
Brain:	Auditory and visual hallucinations, as well as arousing auditory and visual memories	x	x							x	
Brain:	Loss of a sense of body position, or body image. Such blurring, or total loss of the sense of body image and body position, may even result in a disintegration of all sense of space and self, causing affected people to feel a sense of being 'one with the universe', of depersonalization, or out-of-body		x								

Symptoms of hypoxia		Hypoxia	Hypoxia	Hypoxia	Anemia	Sleep apnea	Altitude sickness	Altitude sickness	Chronic mountain sickness	Carbon monoxide poisoning	Carbon monoxide poisoning
	experiences										
Brain:	Confusion								x	x	x
Brain:	Dementia									delayed	
Brain:	Loss of consciousness, together with abnormal breathing / respiratory arrest; death			x						x	
Brain:	Impaired alertness					x					
Brain:	Poor concentration				x						
Central Nervous System:	Slower reaction time					x					
Ear:	Tinnitus (perception of sound within the human ear in the absence of corresponding external sound)								x		
Sleep:	Sleep disturbance, insomnia					x	x	x	x		
Sleep:	Sleep Paralysis, a condition in which the sufferer partially awakes, and yet is still dreaming, those dreams are always nightmares, typically a presence of some sort of horrifying entity.					x					
Sleep:	Daytime sleepiness					x					
Sleep:	Somnolence (drowsiness, a state of near-sleep, a strong desire for sleep)						x	x			
Motor:	Muscle tremors, ataxia, in-coordination with diminished hand-eye coordination. Initiation of movements and actual movement requires enormous mental effort.	x									
Motor:	Intermittent claudication of the legs (limping)				very severe						
Motor:	Unsteady or strange gait (walking)									x, delayed	
Motor:	Parkinson's disease-like syndromes									delayed	
Vision:	Eye yellowing				x						

Symptoms of hypoxia		Hypoxia	Hypoxia	Hypoxia	Anemia	Sleep apnea	Altitude sickness	Altitude sickness	Chronic mountain sickness	Carbon monoxide poisoning	Carbon monoxide poisoning
Vision:	Vision problems					x					
Vision:	Narrowing of the visual fields resulting in tunnel vision as well as blurring of vision. This is the "tunnel experience" reported by those reporting near death experiences.	x									
Vision:	Failure of the entire retina, total loss of vision, cortical blindness		x							delayed	
Skin:	Cyanosis: blue coloration of the skin and tongue due to desaturation of hemoglobin	x							x		
Skin:	Paresthesia / "Pins and needles"						x	x			
Liver:	Liver function impairment, particularly fatty liver diseases					x					
Spleen:	Enlarged spleen				x						
Eating:	Anorexia								x		
Eating:	Lack of appetite						x	x			
Eating:	Nausea or vomiting						x	x		x	x
Eating:	Pica (consumption of non-food items such as soil, paper, wax, grass, ice, and hair)				iron deficiency						
Intestinal:	Changed stool color				x						
Muscular:	Fatigue or weakness				x	x	x	x	x	x	
Skin:	Skin paleness				x						
Skin:	Skin yellowing				x						
Skin:	Skin coldness				x						
General:	General malaise (a feeling of general discomfort or uneasiness)				x		x	x		x	
Oedema:	Peripheral oedema (swelling of hands, feet, and face)						x	x			
Oedema:	Pulmonary edema (fluid in the lungs): Symptoms similar to bronchitis, Persistent dry cough, Fever, Shortness of breath even when resting							x			
Oedema:	Cerebral edema (swelling of the brain): Headache that does not respond to analgesics, Unsteady gait, Gradual loss of consciousness, Increased nausea, Retinal hemorrhage							x			

5.4. HYPOGLYCEMIA: LOW BLOOD GLUCOSE

Hypoglycemia is an abnormally low content of glucose in the blood. Depletion of sugar in blood and glycogen reservoirs causes tiredness. When the heart- and breathing rate is rapid you will use glucose and glycogen for fast energy supply instead of the slow fat burning. This will deplete your small reservoirs of glucose and glycogen.

5.5. TYRAMINE

Tyramine acts as a releasing agent for catecholamines (dopamine, norepinephrine (noradrenaline), epinephrine (adrenaline)). http://en.wikipedia.org/wiki/Tyramine

Tyramine gives the adrenaline "cheese effect".
- High blood pressure,
- Headache,
- Heart pounding and palpitations and
- The complications included subarachnoid hemorrhage, hemiplegia, intracranial hemorrhage, cardiac arrhythmias, cardiac failure, pulmonary edema, and death.

Source: Rao 2009.

5.6. MAST CELL DEGRANULATION

During mast cell degranulation not only histamine is released but other mediators as well. Every mediator has its typical symptoms. (Table 8). Because so many different mediators are involved this list of possible symptoms is also large (Table 8, Table 9, Table 10, Table 11).

Table 8 Mast cell derived mediators considered to contribute substantially to the clinical symptoms and manifestations of Mast Cell Activation (Valent 2012)

Mediator	Symptom(s)/sign(s)	Consensus level[1]
Histamine	headache, hypotension, urticaria with or without angioedema, pruritus, diarrhea	95%
PGD_2	mucus secretion, bronchoconstriction, vascular instability	95%
PAF[2]	abdominal cramping, pulmonary edema, urticaria, bronchoconstriction, hypotension, arrythmia	90%
Proinflammatory cytokines	local inflammation, edema formation, leukocyte migration	80%
LTC_4 and LTD_4	mucus secretion, edema formation, vascular instability	80%
Chemokines	acute inflammation and leukocyte recruitment, leukocyte migration	70%
Tryptase	endothelial activation with consecutive inflammatory reactions	65%

PAF = Platelet-activating factor; LT = leukotriene.

[1] Percentage of members agreeing that these mediators play a predominant role in clinical signs and symptoms recorded in patients with MCA.

[2] Evidence for a role of platelet-activating factor as a potential mediator of urticaria stems primarily from data obtained from healthy volunteers and in vitro studies.

Table 9 Symptoms significantly associated with Mastocytosis (Hermine 2008)

Previously identified symptoms[a]	Symptoms not previously reported
Fatigue (asthenia)	Food and drug allergy/intolerance
Anaphylaxis	Muscle/joint pain and cramps
Sweating	Aerophagia/eruction
Flushing	Reduced sexual relations
Pruritus	Ocular discomfort
Erythemateous crises	Tinnitus
Epigastric pain	Pseudo-occlusive syndrome
Diarrhea	Infections (bronchitis, rhinitis, and conjunctivitis)
Dyspnea/bronchoreactivity	Olfactive intolerance
Nausea/vomiting	Reduced mobility
Bone pain	Hemorrhoidal inflammation
Headache	Cough
Memory loss	Ear/nose/throat inflammation
Difficulty with social interactions	General pain
Reduced performance status	
Depression	

Table 10 Signs and symptoms of patients with Mast Cell Activation Syndrome (Hamilton 2011)

Sign or symptom	Total (%), n = 18
Abdominal pain	17 (94)
Dermatographism	16 (89)
Flushing	16 (89)
Headache	15 (83)
Poor concentration and memory	12 (67)
Diarrhea	12 (67)
Naso-ocular	7 (39)
Asthma	7 (39)
Anaphylaxis	3 (17)

Table 11 Top 20 symptoms (symptoms which were mentioned most frequent) in a 2010 survey of mastocytosis patients (König, 2011)

1	Pruritus (itch)
2	Fatigue
3	Skin lesions
4	Bone pain
5	Headache
6	Tachycardia (fast heart beat)
7	Joint pain
8	Flushing
9	Diarrhoea
10	Sleeping problems
11	Dizziness
12	Concentration problems
13	Gastrointestinal tract problems
14	Nausea
15	Muscle pain
16	Abdominal pain
17	Memory problems
18	Drowsiness
19	Skin reddening
20	Shortness of breath

6. INDIVIDUAL SYMPTOMS

6.1. DIARRHEA, CONSTIPATION, IRRITABLE BOWEL

"The main complaints of patients with Irritable bowel syndrome (IBS, or spastic colon) are chronic abdominal pain, discomfort, bloating, and alteration of bowel habits. Diarrhea or constipation may predominate, or they may alternate (classified as IBS-D, IBS-C or IBS-A, respectively). The primary symptoms of IBS are abdominal pain or discomfort in association with frequent diarrhea or constipation, a change in bowel habits. There may also be urgency for bowel movements, a feeling of incomplete evacuation (tenesmus), bloating or abdominal distention. In some cases, the symptoms are relieved by bowel movements.
People with IBS, more commonly than others, have
- *gastroesophageal reflux,*
- *fibromyalgia,*
- *backache,*
- *depression,*
- *headache,*
- *anxiety,*
- *chronic fatigue syndrome."*

Source: http://en.wikipedia.org/wiki/Irritable_bowel_syndrome

✓ Investigate if you suffer from histamine intolerance and/or mast cell activation.

6.2. ACID/GASTROESOPHAGEAL REFLUX, GERD

"Gastroesophageal reflux disease (GERD), gastro-oesophageal reflux disease (GORD), gastric reflux disease, or acid reflux disease is a chronic symptom of mucosal damage caused by stomach acid coming up from the stomach into the esophagus.
Gastric H2 receptor blockers (such as ranitidine, famotidine and cimetidine) can reduce gastric secretion of acid. These drugs are technically antihistamines. They relieve complaints in about 50% of all GERD patients."
Source: http://en.wikipedia.org/wiki/Gastroesophageal_reflux_disease

✓ When H2 histamine receptor blockers relieve complaints of GERD investigate if you suffer from histamine intolerance and/or mast cell activation.

6.3. DYSMENORRHOEA

The uterine endometrium contains mast cells and they are proposed to play an important role in embryo implantation. The female hormones estradiol and progesterone attract mast cells to the uterus and provoke their maturation and degranulation (Jensen 2010). "Once the lining of the uterus starts breaking down, as it does at the start of every period, the body naturally releases histamines with severe cramps as a result. The histamine released also causes water retention and a temporary weight gain."

"Molecular compounds called prostaglandins are released during menstruation, due to the destruction of the endometrial cells, and the resultant release of their contents. Release of prostaglandins and other inflammatory mediators in the uterus cause the uterus to contract. These substances are thought to be a major factor in primary dysmenorrhea. When the uterine muscles contract, they constrict the blood supply to the tissue of the endometrium, which, in turn, breaks down and dies. These uterine contractions continue as they squeeze the old, dead endometrial tissue through the cervix and out of the body through the vagina. These contractions, and the resulting temporary oxygen deprivation to nearby tissues, are responsible for the pain or "cramps" experienced during menstruation."
Source: http://en.wikipedia.org/wiki/Dysmenorrhea

6.4. ARTHRITIS

Mediators released by mast cell degranalation may cause inflammation of joints (Nigrovic 2004).

6.5. FIBROMYALGIA

"The main complaint of patients with the Fibromyalgia Syndrome is pain. It is a syndrome meaning that the underlying cause is unknown.
Signs and symptoms
The defining symptoms of fibromyalgia are chronic widespread pain, fatigue, and heightened pain in response to tactile pressure (allodynia). Other symptoms may include tingling of the skin, prolonged muscle spasms, weakness in the limbs, nerve pain, muscle twitching, palpitations, functional bowel disturbances, and chronic sleep disturbances.
Many patients experience cognitive dysfunction (known as "fibrofog"), which may be characterized by impaired concentration, problems with short and long-term memory, short-term memory consolidation, impaired speed of performance, inability to multi-task, cognitive overload, and diminished attention span. Fibromyalgia is often associated with anxiety and depressive symptoms.
Other symptoms often attributed to fibromyalgia that may possibly be due to a comorbid disorder include myofascial pain syndrome, also referred to

as chronic myofascial pain, diffuse non-dermatomal paresthesias, functional bowel disturbances and irritable bowel syndrome, genitourinary symptoms and interstitial cystitis, dermatological disorders, headaches, myoclonic twitches, and symptomatic hypoglycemia. Although fibromyalgia is classified based on the presence of chronic widespread pain, pain may also be localized in areas such as the shoulders, neck, low back, hips, or other areas. Many sufferers also experience varying degrees of myofascial pain and have high rates of comorbid temporomandibular joint disorder. 20–30% of patients with rheumatoid arthritis and systemic lupus erythematosus may also have fibromyalgia."
Source: http://en.wikipedia.org/wiki/Fibromyalgia

✓ Investigate if you suffer from histamine intolerance and/or mast cell activation.

6.6. CYCLIC VOMITING

"Cyclic vomiting syndrome is a condition whose symptoms are recurring attacks of intense nausea, vomiting and sometimes abdominal pain and/or headaches or migraines."
Source: http://en.wikipedia.org/wiki/Cyclic_vomiting_syndrome

Paul (2012) showed that a low-amine diet helped in reducing the symptoms of CVS.

✓ Investigate if you suffer from histamine intolerance and/or mast cell activation.

6.7. HEADACHE AND MIGRAINE

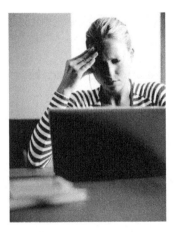

The most common types of headache are the "primary headache disorders", such as tension-type headache and migraine.
http://en.wikipedia.org/wiki/Headache

Cascade proposed by de Wild-Scholten:

Histamine → hypoxia → tension-type headache, aura → adrenaline → vasoconstriction → migraine.

Painkillers
Certain painkillers are DAO enzyme inhibitors or act as mast cell degranulators (Table 13).They may kill the pain initially but they may contribute to the overload of histamine, making your problems worse.

Preventive medicines

"In general, any patient who has frequent headaches or migraine attacks should be considered as a potential candidate for preventive medications instead of being encouraged to take more and more painkillers or other rebound-causing medications. Preventive medications are taken on a daily basis. Some patients may require preventive medications for many years; others may require them for only a relatively short period of time such as six months. Effective preventive medications have been found to come from many classes of medications including neuronal stabilizing agents (aka anticonvulsants), antidepressants, <u>antihypertensives</u>, and <u>antihistamines</u>. Some effective preventive medications include Elavil (amitriptyline), Depakote (valproate), Topamax (topiramate), and Inderal (propranolol)."
http://en.wikipedia.org/wiki/Medication_overuse_headache

Medicines which block the action of histamine (histamine receptor antagonists = antihistamines) and/or adrenaline (adrenergic receptor antagonists) prevent the histamine cascade of symptoms.
The antidepressants amitriptyline (tricyclic) acts primarily as a serotonin-norepinephrine reuptake inhibitor. It *additionally* functions as a H1-, H2- and H4- histamine, α1-adrenergic receptor antagonist!
http://en.wikipedia.org/wiki/Amitriptyline
The antihypertensive propranolol is a beta-blocker so blocking the beta-adrenergic receptors.

- ✓ When anti-histamines are effective investigate if you suffer from histamine intolerance and/or mast cell activation.
- ✓ When you suffer from hypertension investigate if you suffer from hypoxia.

Magnesium, L-carnitine

- ▪ *"Oral supplementation with magnesium oxide and L-carnitine and concurrent supplementation of Mg-L-carnitine besides routine treatments could be effective in migraine prophylaxis"* (Tarighat Esfanjani 2012).
- ▪ *"Considering these features of magnesium, the fact that magnesium deficiency may be present in up to half of migraine patients, and that routine blood tests are not indicative of magnesium status, empiric treatment with at least oral magnesium is warranted in all migraine sufferers."* (Mauskop 2012)

Magnesium is a mast cell stabilizer. Could L-carnitine act as a methyldonor in the conversion of histamine to methylhistamine? The fact that magnesium and L-carnitine are used to treat migraine patient is an indication that migraine could be caused by histamine intolerance and/or mast cell degranulation.

Hypoxia

Migraine was provoked in six (42%) migraine patients by hypoxia and the median time to attacks was 5 hours (Schoonman 2006).

Brain damage

Migraine patients show ischemic lesions in the brain (Palm-Meinders 2012). It is likely that the lesions are the result of insufficient oxygen supply (hypoxia).

6.8. CHRONIC FATIGUE

The main complaint of patients with the Chronique Fatigue Syndrome (CFS) is tiredness.

"Primary symptoms
The fatigue of CFS is accompanied by characteristic illness symptoms lasting at least 6 months. These symptoms include:

- *increased malaise (extreme exhaustion and sickness) following physical activity or mental exertion*
- *problems with sleep*
- *difficulties with memory and concentration*
- *persistent muscle pain*
- *joint pain (without redness or swelling)*
- *headache*
- *tender lymph nodes in the neck or armpit*
- *sore throat*

Other Symptoms
The symptoms listed above are the symptoms used to diagnose CFS. However, many CFS patients and patients in general may experience other symptoms, including:

- *brain fog (feeling like you're in a mental fog)*
- *difficulty maintaining an upright position, dizziness, balance problems or fainting*
- *allergies or sensitivities to foods, odors, chemicals, medications, or noise*
- *irritable bowel*
- *chills and night sweats*
- *visual disturbances (sensitivity to light, blurring, eye pain)*
- *depression or mood problems (irritability, mood swings, anxiety, panic attacks)"*

Source: CDC in the US http://www.cdc.gov/cfs/symptoms/index.html

✓ Investigate if you suffer from histamine intolerance and/or mast cell activation.

7. DIAGNOSIS

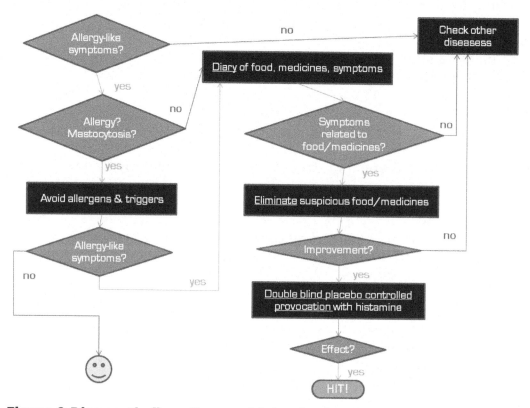

Figure 9 Diagnostic flow diagram histamine intolerance

7.1. YOUR MEDICAL HISTORY

What are your symptoms? Since when? How often?
What are your triggers of symptoms?
What medicines do you take?
What other diseases do you have?

7.2. CHECK FOR OTHER DISEASES

- **Allergies**: excessive activation of mast cells and basophils by a type of antibody called Immunoglobulin E (IgE).
- **Mastocytosis**: the presence of too many mast cells.
- **Inflammatory Bowel Diseases (IBD)** like Crohn's disease and Ulcerative Colitis.
- **Infection with Helicobacter pylori**
- **Lactose intolerance**: insufficient levels of lactase, the enzyme that metabolizes lactose into glucose and galactose
- **Fructose malabsorption:** impaired absorption of fructose by deficient fructose carriers in the small intestine's enterocytes. This results in an increased concentration of fructose in the entire intestine
- **Coeliac disease:** an autoimmune disorder of the small intestine caused by a reaction to gliadin, a gluten protein found in wheat

- **Hereditary fructose intolerance:** an inborn error of fructose metabolism caused by a deficiency of the enzyme aldolase B
- **Vitamin B6 deficiency**.
- **Leaky gut**
- **Intestinal mucosal disorders**: for example fluorouracil anti-cancer drugs (Goto 2011, Namikawa 2012)

7.3.   DIARY

For a few weeks write down what & when you eat and drink, other possible triggers, what medicines you take and which symptoms you have and when. It is important to write down the times so you will be able to find out the delay with which you experience your symptoms.
In Appendix 1 a diary template is provided.
When keeping your diary try to measure or have measured your blood pressure and pulse a few times. Normal blood pressure is 120/80.

7.4.   ELIMINATION DIET

Eliminate the food that is rich in histamine, other biogenic amines, mast cell degranulators and substances which decrease the activity of the enzymes. Continue to write in your diary. When you see a significant reduction in symptoms you may be suffering from histamine intolerance and/or mast cell activation.

7.5.   HISTAMINE SKIN PRICK TEST

People with histamine intolerance have a lower degradation rate of histamine. In the histamine skin prick test the size of the wheal is measured 50 minutes after pricking with a 1% histamine solution. The wheal is larger in patients with histamine intolerance (Kofler 2011). Everybody who performs skin prick tests is able to perform a histamine prick test. You just have to wait for a longer time.

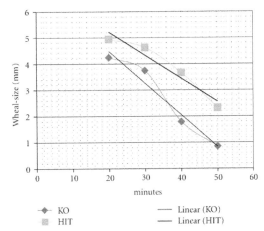

Figure 10 Wheal size and time course of histamine-wheal in the control-group and the HIT group; measured at 20, 30, 40 and 50 minutes. Control group = 75, HIT group = 81 (Kofler 2011)

7.6. DAO ACTIVITY IN BLOOD SERUM

SCiOTEC in Austria provides test kits of activity of the enzyme DAO in *serum or plasma* (D-HIT). The correlation between DAO-activity and symptoms is shown in Figure 11.

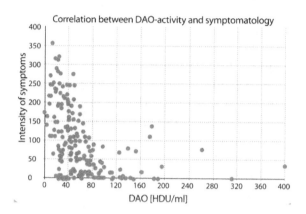

Figure 11 Correlation between DAO-activity and HIT symptomatology (Sciotec D-HIT product data sheet), HDU = Histamine Degrading Units

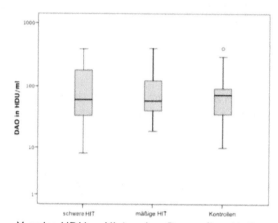

Y-axis: HDU = Histamine Degrading Units,
X-axis: heavy HIT, moderate HIT, Controls

Figure 12 DAO-activity in *serum* of HIT patients and controls (Töndury 2008).

Töndury 2008 concluded (Figure 12): "*Based on the patient's history with allergy like symptoms occurring with intake of histamine rich food, determination of DAO activity in the serum does not facilitate diagnosis of HIT in routine clinical practice.*"

Kofler 2009 concluded: "*A correlation between DAO-concentration and clinical diagnosis is not reproducible. We think therefore that the determination of DAO does not provide help to diagnose histamine intolerance.*"

DAO activity in *blood serum or plasma* is not representative for the DAO activity in the *small intestine* which is the most important location of histamine degradation.

✓ DAO activity testing in blood is not recommended.

7.7. DOUBLE-BLIND PLACEBO-CONTROLLED ORAL PROVOCATION

Double-blind, placebo-controlled oral provocation (DBPCOP) with a non-toxic dose of 75 mg histamine provoked symptoms in half of the healthy (!) volunteers (Wöhrl 2004).
  ✓ DBPCOP with histamine is not recommended for diagnosis purposes.

7.8. GENE TESTING

Zentrum für Nephrologie und Stoffwechsel Dr. Mato Nagel (Weißwasser, Germany) is performing a **DAO** gen test on a blood sample. The price is 250 euro for the complete gen (status 27-2-2013).
http://www.moldiag.de/de/gen/104610.htm

Novogenia GmbH is currently performing a **HNMT**-study to investigate the correlation between various defects in the HNMT gene and symptoms of histamine intolerance. The test is done on a saliva sample. The price is 228 euro including VAT (status 27-2-2013).
http://novogenia.com/studien/hnmt-histamineintolerance-english/

7.9. MAST CELL ACTIVATION SYNDROME

Proposed criteria for Mast Cell Activation Syndrome (MCAS) (In: Frieri 2012; from Akin 2010):

---

1. Episodic _symptoms_ consistent with mast cell mediator release affecting ≥ 2 organ systems evidenced as follows:
   a. Skin: urticaria, angioedema, flushing
   b. Gastrointestinal: nausea, vomiting, diarrhea, abdominal cramping
   c. Cardiovascular: hypotensive syncope or near syncope, tachycardia
   d. Respiratory: wheezing
   e. Naso-ocular: conjunctival injection, pruritus, nasal stuffiness
2. A _decrease_ in the frequency or severity or resolution _of symptoms with antimediator therapy_: H1- and H2-histamine receptor inverse agonists, antileukotriene medications (cysteinyl leukotriene receptor blockers or 5-lipoxygenase inhibitor), or mast cell stabilizers (cromolyn sodium).
3. Evidence of an _increase in_ a validated urinary or serum _marker of mast cell activation_: documentation of an increase of the marker to greater than the patient's baseline value during a symptomatic period of ≥ 2 occasions or, if baseline tryptase levels are persistently > 15 ng, documentation of an increase in tryptase level above baseline value on 1 occasion. Total serum tryptase level is recommended as the mark of choice; less specific (also from basophils) are 24-h urinary metabolites of PGD2 (Prostaglandin D2) or its metabolite 11-β-prostaglandin F2.
4. _Rule out primary and secondary causes of mast cell activation_ and well defined clinical idiopathic entities.

MCAS for now remains an idiopathic disorder; however in some cases, it could be an early reflection of a monoclonal population of mast cells, in which case with time it could meet the criteria for MMAS (Monoclonal Mast Cell Activation Syndrome) as 1 or 2 minor criteria for mastocytosis are fulfilled.

---

8. TREATMENT OF HISTAMINE INTOLERANCE & MAST CELL ACTIVATION

With the treatment we like to prevent *unnecessary* activation of our defence system. We must be careful however not to harm or block this system since we need it when we have an infection.

The aim of the treatment is to:
1. prevent a leaky gut,
2. prevent overloading the enzymes,
3. prevent mast cell degranulation,
4. prevent the effect of histamine, and

Discuss the steps you like to take with your health professional.
A dietician can help with the interpretation of the diary and advise on keeping a well balanced diet which has all necessary nutrients.

After the elimination diet it is time to add one-by-one each suspicious food and check if this gives symptoms (so-called provocation). Again, write results down in your diary. Every now and then you need to check it again because your sensitivity may change over time. Remember that the symptoms are dose dependent. You need to find out your personal threshold by modifying the amounts consumed.
Unfortunately there is no legal obligation to indicate the histamine concentration on food labels!
See Appendix for food lists.

General tips
- ✓ Grow your own herbs, vegetables and fruit.
- ✓ Buy and use fresh (frozen) ingredients.
- ✓ Buy unminced meat.
- ✓ Buy local and seasonal food which has less chance of degradation and is better from an environmental point of view.
- ✓ Buy organic/eco food which has no or less food additives and pesticides.
- ✓ Transport your fresh ingredients in a cool bag.
- ✓ Eat regular and small amounts to avoid overloading your enzymes.

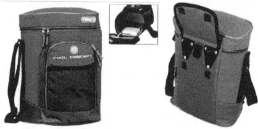

Figure 13 Norlander bike cool bag Deluxe

Foods most frequently reported (Jarisch):

Alcoholic beverages (especially red wine)

Cheese (especially hard cheeses like Emmental cheese)

Chocolate

Cured sausages (Salami etc.)

Nuts

Tomatoes

Strawberries, **citrus fruits** and other histamine liberators

Sauerkraut

Spinach

Fish

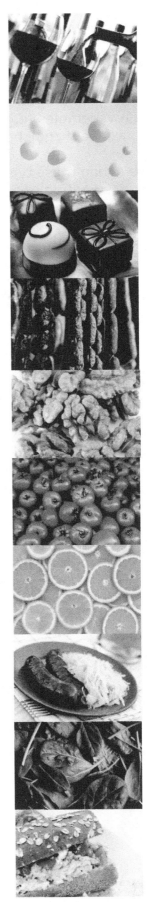

8.1. PREVENT LEAKY GUT

8.1.1. Deactivate lectins in food

Foods rich in lectins are legumes (e.g. beans, lentils, peas, peanuts), grains (e.g. wheat) and nightshade vegetables (e.g. potatoes, tomatoes, eggplant, wolfberry/goji berry).

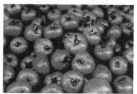

✓ Before eating these types of foods deactivate the lectins by cooking, soaking, sprouting or fermenting.

8.2. PREVENT ENZYME OVERLOAD

8.2.1. Fresh proteins

Proteins degrade to histamine and other biogenic amines.
Histidine-rich food has the highest *potential* to degrade to histamine-rich food (Table 25).

Cheese
Results of the European project BIAMFOOD (Lolkema 2011):
"Histamine levels were found to be higher in cheeses from raw than from pasteurized milk, in processed than in unprocessed cheeses, and in long ripening cheeses. The highest histamine content was detected in commercial blue cheese samples."

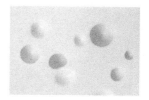

Fish
Tuna, mackerel and anchovies are rich in histidine. Bacteria in the gut of the fish convert histidine to histamine. The longer the fish stays with its gut the higher the concentration of histamine.

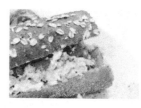

Meat
Minced meat has a higher surface area and degrades faster. The meat of sausages is not fresh.

Vegetables
Eggplant, Sauerkraut and spinach can be high in histamine.

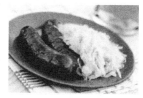

Tips
- ✓ Buy cheese from pasteurized milk.
- ✓ Buy cheeses with short ripening.
- ✓ Eat fresh fish.
- ✓ Select fish low in histidine.
- ✓ Select non-minced meat.

8.2.2. Avoid bacteria which convert histidine to histamine

See (Table 2).

When a health professional proposes **antibiotics** because of a suspected bacterial inflammation request that the *bacterial infection* is proven by making a culture! Inflammation may be the result of non-bacterial causes. After the use of antibiotics your may end up with wrong gut bacteria.

8.2.3. Avoid inhibitors of DAO- , MAO-, HNMT-enzyme

Avoid medicines which are:
- Inhibitors of the enzymes DAO, MAO and HNMT,
- Vitamin B6 antagonists (Table 13).

Warning: do not change your medicines without consulting your health professional!

8.2.4. Histamine destroyers
✓ **Vitamin C**

"In the March 2011 "Journal of Evidence-Based Complementary & Alternative Medicine," researchers reported that Vitamin C works as an antihistamine by destroying the molecular structure of the imidole ring of the histamine molecule, thereby decreasing the amount of histamine in the blood." http://www.livestrong.com/article/444603-antihistamine-action-of-vitamin-c/

8.2.5. DAO enzyme

Figure 14 shows that the supplementation of DAO leads to a statistically significant reduction of histamine-associated symptoms (Komericki 2010).

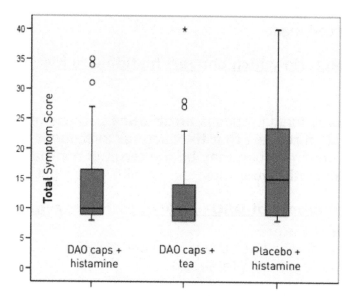

Figure 14 Total symptom score after double blind, placebo controlled oral provocation with 75 mg pure histamine conducted in four Austrian Medical Centres (Missbichler 2010, Komericki 2010)

DAO capsules are provided under the names of DAOSiN (from SCiOTEC) and histame.
Long-term effects are unknown. Consult your health professional first!

8.3. PREVENT MAST CELL DEGRANULATION

8.3.1. Mast cell stabilizers

Mast cell stabilizers prevent the degranulation of mast cells.

Mast cell stabilizers in food:
- ✓ **Magnesium** (Kraeuter 1980). Green leafy vegetables are high in magnesium because of the chlorophyll which has magnesium in the centre of its molecule.

Mast cell stabilizing medicines are:
- ▪ **Cromoglicic acid**, marketed as sodium cromoglicate (Nalcrom). Take 15 minutes before eating.
- ▪ **Ketotifen**, also a H1-anti-histamine.

Consult your health professional!

8.3.2. Avoid mast cell degranulators

✓ See list in paragraph 4.5. The name "mast cell degranulator" is preferred over the term "histamine liberator" because not only histamine is liberated but also may other mediators.

✓ See Food lists in Appendix. From the cited references it is unclear on what the qualification of histamine liberator is based on, so there is a high uncertainty here.

✓ **Avoid fragrances/aromas**

Acetaldehyde is a mast cell degranulator. It has the smell of apple. Major sources of exposure are from the oxidation of ethanol after drinking alcohol and from tobacco smoking. Other sources are cosmetic products and from burning of fossil fuels. In foods it is present naturally or it is added as flavorant. The content of acetaldehyde in food does not need to be indicated on the label. The estimated exposure for food groups in decreasing order are: alcohol-free-beverages, fruits (content increases with ripening), milk products, bread, vegetables, jams (Uebelacker 2011). See Table 20.

The mast cell degranulator effect of vinegar could be due to acetaldehyde (incomplete conversion to acetic acid).

Spices and herbs
Spices and herbs contain several fragrances (Table 19).

Fruit
Citrus fruit *peel* contains limonene, citral, linalool and geraniol (Table 19).

Chocolate
The two main classes of odorant compounds in chocolate are pyrazines and aldehydes. Compounds in dark chocolate which are established contact allergens according to "Opinion on fragrance allergens in cosmetic products, European Commission 2012" are benzyl alcohol, linalool, benzaldehyde and vanillin (Counet 2002).

Wine
"Some of the identified aroma compounds include the following:(Robinson 2006) Methoxypyrazine-grassy, herbaceous aroma compound associated with Cabernet Sauvignon and Sauvignon blanc. Monoterpenes-responsible for the floral aromatics of varieties like Gewürztraminer, Muscat and Riesling. Includes geraniol, linalool and nerol. Norisoprenoids-Carotenoid derived aromatic compounds[6] that includes megastigmatrienone which produces some of the spice notes associated with Chardonnay and zingerone responsible for the different spice notes associated with Syrah. Other norisoprenoids include raspberry ketone which produces some of the raspberry aromas associated with red wine, damascenone which produces some of the rose oil aromas associated with Pinot noir and vanillin. Thiols-sulfur contain compounds that can produce an aroma of garlic and onion that is considered a wine fault (mercaptans). They have also been found to contribute to some of the varietal aromas associated with Cabernet Sauvignon, Gewürztraminer, Merlot, Muscat, Petit Manseng, Pinot blanc, Pinot gris, Riesling, Scheurebe, Semillon and Sylvaner."
http://en.wikipedia.org/wiki/Aroma_of_wine#Identified_aroma_compounds

✓ **Fresh lipids**

Lipid degradation leads to hydrolysis- and oxidation products.

Unsaturated fatty acids (oleic acid, linoleic acid, alpha-linolenic acid, eicosapentaenoic acid, docosahexaenoic acid) have one or more double bonds between carbon atoms and hydrolyse in the presence of water or oxidize in the presence of oxygen. Heat or light accelerates oxidation. Anti-oxidants prevent oxidation. Lipids high in polyunsaturated fatty acid have the highest risk to become rancid. Volatile oxidation products are released like aldehydes and ketones some of those may cause mast cell degranulation!
However healthier dietary fats are the monounsaturated fat and polyunsaturated fat... Also some unsaturated fats are essential. To conclude: we must eat fresh lipids.
Table 21 shows the lipid content of some foods.

Essential fatty acids
"Fatty acids that are required by the human body but cannot be made in sufficient quantity from other substrates, and therefore must be obtained from food, are called essential fatty acids. There are two series of essential fatty acids: one has a double bond three carbon atoms removed from the methyl end; the other has a double bond six carbon atoms removed from the methyl end. Humans lack the ability to introduce double bonds in fatty acids beyond carbons 9 and 10, as counted from the carboxylic acid side. Two essential fatty acids are <u>linoleic acid (LA)</u> and <u>alpha-linolenic acid (ALA)</u>. They are widely distributed in plant oils. The human body has a limited ability to convert ALA into the longer-chain n-3 fatty acids <u>eicosapentaenoic acid (EPA) and docosahexaenoic acid (DHA)</u>, which can also be obtained from fish." http://en.wikipedia.org/wiki/Fatty_acid

Nuts
"Oils of pecan and pistachio were the most stable, whereas oils of pine nut and walnut were the least stable of the tree nuts almond, Brazil nut, hazelnut, pecan, pine nut, pistachio, and walnut" (Miraliakbari 2008). This could explain the fact that nuts and especially walnuts appear on lists of "histamine liberators".

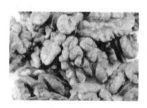

Seeds
Sunflower seeds have a high content of polyunsaturated fatty acids which explains the listing as a "histamine liberator".

Oils
Coconut oil is the oil with least amount of polyunsaturated fatty acids.

Grains, cereals
Oat cereals have the highest amount of polyunsaturated fatty acid and have the highest risk to develop rancidity (Lehtinen 2003).

Chocolate
Poor quality chocolate has a lower cocoa solids percentage and use hydrogenated vegetable oil (trans-fat) instead of cocoa butter. White chocolate has no cocoa solids and is made from a minimum of 20% cocoa butter. Milk chocolate may go rancid due to the fats in the milk going rancid.

Dairy
"Homogenization markedly increases the resistance of milks to oxidized flavor." http://drinc.ucdavis.edu/dairyp/dairyp3.htm

Tips
- ✓ Buy products in opaque packaging, dark bottles and in small quantities.
- ✓ Buy *cold* pressed oils.
- ✓ Buy fresh or homogenized milk.
- ✓ Store nuts and oils dark, dry and cool.
- ✓ Use a vacuum wine saver tool (Vacu Vin) to close opened oil bottles
- ✓ Eat nuts separate and not added to foods like bread and pastes.

✓ Avoid salicylates
When you do not tolerate acetylsalicylic acid (aspirin) you probably have a salicylate sensitivity and you need to avoid salicylates in food (Table 29).
- *"Most fruits, especially berry fruits and dried fruits, contain salicylate.*
- *Vegetables show a wide range from 0 to 6 mg salicylate per 100 g food (for gherkins).*
- *Some herbs and spices were found to contain very high amounts per 100 g, e.g., curry powder, paprika, thyme, garam masala, and rosemary.*
- *Among beverages, tea provides substantial amounts of salicylate.*
- *Licorice and peppermint candies and some honeys contain salicylates.*
- *Cereals, meat, fish, and dairy products contain none or negligible amounts."* (Swain 1985).

8.4. PREVENT HISTAMINE EFFECT

8.4.1. Anti-histamines

Anti-histamines do *not* destroy the histamine but just block the histamine receptor. There are four known histamine receptors: H1, H2, H3 and H4. Warning: when you only take anti-histamine to block H1 the histamine will go to H2, H3 or H4-receptors!

8.4.2. Avoid vasodilators

Histamine lowers the blood pressure by vasodilation. Various foods and medicines also cause vasodilation so if you have a hypotension it is best to avoid them.

Examples of vasodilators are:
- Ethanol (alcohol),
- Theobromine (in cocoa, chocolate, tea plant Camellia sinensis),
- Capsaicin (in chili peppers),
- Papaverine (in the opium poppy Papaver somniferum)
- Estrogen,
- Nitric oxide (NO in air pollution),
- Nitrites (in poppers and anti-hypertensive medicines).

Source: http://en.wikipedia.org/wiki/Vasodilation

✓ **Avoid Nitrites/Nitrates in food**

Cured sausages almost always have nitrites/nitrates added. Some vegetables can be high in nitrate for example spinach and red beetroot (Table 23).

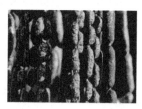

8.5. FINDING GOOD RECIPES

Finding good recipes without the bad ingredients can be quite a challenge! Special recipe books are available for sufferers of histamine intolerance but since everybody has their own sensitivity it is difficult to make a selection of recipes which are tolerated by all sufferers.

- ✓ Leave the undesired ingredients out and see if the compromise is acceptable.
- ✓ On a few recipe websites you can search for recipes and select ingredients you *don't* want, for example http://allrecipes.com/
- ✓ For family members who do not suffer from histamine intolerance or mast cell activation it is possible in many cases to serve the bad ingredient separate.
- ✓ Find inspiration on: http://thelowhistaminechef.com/

9. TREATMENT OF HYPOXIA

To decrease the risk of developing hypoxia a few tips:

- **Optimize your level of hemoglobin**, especially vegetarians and women with menorrhagia (abnormally heavy and prolonged menstrual period).
- **Ventilate your room continuously** to let oxygen in and carbon dioxide out.
- **Avoid fireplaces** because they consume oxygen and if not operated well may produce carbon monoxide.
- **Avoid regions with air pollution** (especially carbon monoxide and nitrogen oxide).
  US Air Now: http://www.airnow.gov/,
  UK Air: http://uk-air.defra.gov.uk/latest/ ,
  U.S Embassy Beijing Air Quality Monitor: http://beijing.usembassy-china.org.cn/070109air.html,
  U.S. Consulate Shanghai Air Quality Monitor:
  http://shanghai.usembassy-china.org.cn/airmonitor.html.
- **Select a living area with low carbon monoxide and low nitrogen oxide concentrations** (Nattero 1996).
- **Avoid cigarette smoke**.
- **Do not eat/drink before going to sleep** because digestion consumes oxygen.
- **No plants in your sleeping room** because they consume oxygen at night.
- **Do your physical exercises in fresh air in the aerobic regime.** Avoid anaerobic conditions. A pulse oximeter can help you to train in the right regime. Walking for example.
- **Avoid quick visits to high altitudes.** At high altitude the air pressure is lower.
- **Drive an electric car** because it has zero emission!

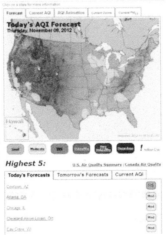

Source: http://www.airnow.gov/

Figure 15 Air quality forecast U.S.A

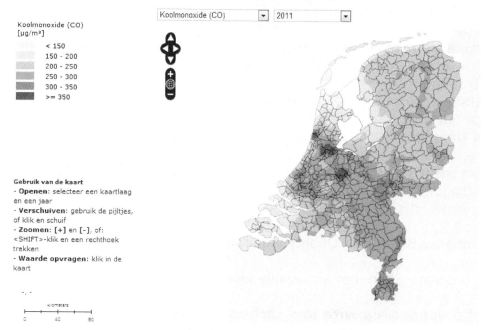

Figure 16 Carbon monoxide concentration map of the Netherlands 2011

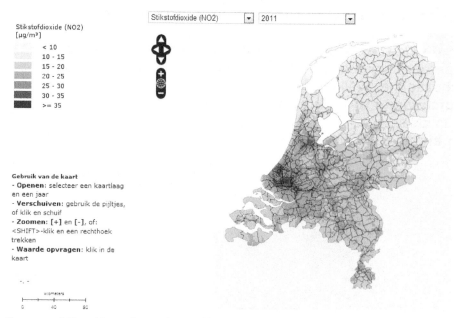

Figure 17 Nitrogen oxide concentration map of the Netherlands 2011

10. TREATMENT OF DYSMENORRHOEA

✓ **Increase oxygen saturation!!** See the chapter about treatment of hypoxia.

✓ **Low estrogen diet**
A low-fat vegetarian diet was associated with reduction in dysmenorrheal duration and intensity. The symptom effects might be mediated by dietary influences on estrogen activity (Barnard 2000).
More estrogen, more mast cells in uterine endometrium, more histamine released during period?

✓ **High omega-3 fatty acid diet**
The prostaglandins derived from marine n-3 fatty acids are normally less aggressive and therefore expected to be associated with milder symptoms. A higher intake of marine n-3 fatty acids correlates with milder menstrual symptoms (Deutch 1995).
Neptune Krill Oil can significantly reduce dysmenorrhea and the emotional symptoms of premenstrual syndrome and is shown to be significantly more effective for the complete management of premenstrual symptoms compared to omega-3 fish oil (Sampalis 2003).
Supplementation with omega-3 fatty acids reduced the symptom intensity of primary dysmenorrhea. Supplementation efficacy was sufficient to decrease the ibuprofen rescue dose (Rahbar 2012).

✓ **Ibuprofen**
Hopefully you can do without ibuprofen when you have implemented the above stated recommendations. Ibuprofen is inhibiting the enzyme cyclooxygenase (COX), which converts arachidonic acid to prostaglandin H2 (PGH2).

11. APP

The medicine and food lists in this book are available as App in the iTunes Store (Apple) and it is called "Histamine Intolerance". http://www.histamine-intolerance.info/app.php . An Android version is planned.

HOME:

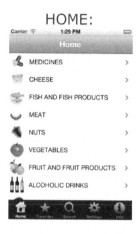

MEDICINE example: CHEESE example:

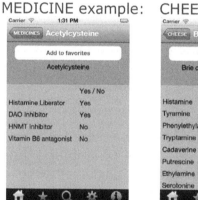
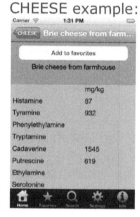

FAVORITES: SEARCH: SETTINGS:

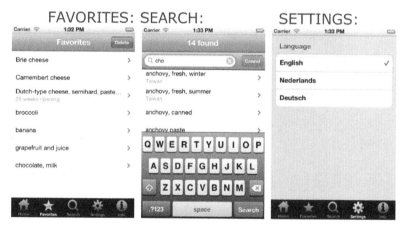

12. SUGGESTIONS FOR RESEARCH

- *Oral* challenge studies on established (fragrance) contact allergens.
- Could a **pheochromocytoma** (tumor of adrenal gland) develop after many years of histamine intolerance?

13. ABOUT THE AUTHOR

Mariska de Wild-Scholten (1964) studied geology at Utrecht University in the Netherlands where she specialized in the chemistry of the earth. Currently, she works as a professional in the field of life cycle assessments (LCA) of photovoltaics to investigate the environmental impacts of the production of photovoltaic systems. She has published many papers on this topic and was invited speaker on several conferences. Since February 2011 she is self-employed consultant on the same topic. Using her expertise on retrieving and judging scientific literature, she was able to find out the triggers for her histamine–related health complaints. This book presents her main findings and is aimed at providing practical knowledge to patients, health professionals, researchers and politicians to increase the general awareness of histamine intolerance.

http://www.histamine-intolerance.info/
http://www.smartgreenscans.nl/

14. ACKNOWLEDGEMENTS

The author would like to thank the patients who were willing to share their history and gave permission to include it in this book.

The open presentation of symptoms and discussions in several Facebook groups is highly appreciated.

Stans van der Poel kindly provided her tool to measure heart- and breathing rates and breathing volume. http://www.stansvanderpoel.nl/

The "Write Your Book in 28 Days" by Nisandeh Neta accelerated the writing and publishing process. http://www.opencircles.nl/

Paul de Wild carefully reviewed the manuscript.

Useful comments to the first edition were received from Dr. Imke Reese (http://www.ernaehrung-allergologie.de/).

Thanx!

APPENDIX 1: DIARY

Table 12 Diary for diagnosis histamine intolerance / mast cell activation
Excel file is available on: http://www.histamine-intolerance.info/

HISTAMINE INTOLERANCE / MAST CELL ACTIVATION DIARY												
Name:												
Day	**Date & time**	**T**	**P**	**Wind speed**	**Wind**	**Rain /Snow**	**Food / Medicine /Trigger**	**Suspicious food / medicine / trigger**	**Symptoms**	**Blood pressure**		
		°C	hPa	m/s	N-E-S-W	mm				Syst (mmHg)	Dia (mmHg)	Pulse

APPENDIX 2: TABLES

Table 13 Medicines which inhibit enzymes or can degranulate mast cells

Name	Detail	DAO inhibitors	Vitamin B6 antagonists	HNMT inhibitors	Mast cell degranulators
* Contrast media *	Contrast media				Lochner2012, Steneberg2007
Acemetacin	NSAID	Lochner2012, Steneberg2007			
Acetylcysteine	Mucolytics	Steneberg2007, Jarisch2004			Lochner2012
Acetylsalicylic acid	Analgesics				Lochner2012, Steneberg2007, Jarisch2004
Acriflavine	Antiseptic	Steneberg2007			
Alcuronium	Muscle relaxants	**Sattler1985**			Lochner2012
Alprenolol	Beta-blocker (Antihypertensive)	Lochner2012			
Ambroxol	Mucolytics	Steneberg2007, Jarisch2004			Lochner2012
Amiloride	Diuretics	**Novotny1994**			
Aminophylline	Bronchodilator	Lochner2012, Jarisch2004			
Amitriptyline	Antidepressants	Lochner2012, Steneberg2007, Jarisch2004			
Amodiaquine	Antimalarial			**Horton2005**	
Amphotericin B	Antibiotics				Lochner2012
Barbiturate	Anesthesia				Lochner2012, Steneberg2007
Cefotiame	Antibiotics	Lochner2012, **Sattler1985**			
Cefuroxime	Antibiotics	**Sattler1985**			
Chloroquine	Antimalarial	Lochner2012, Steneberg2007, Jarisch2004, **Sattler1990**		Lochner2012, **Pacifici1992**	
Chlortetracycline	Antibiotics				Lochner2012
Cimetidine	Histamine H2-receptor antagonists	Steneberg2007, **Wantke1998**			
Clavulanic acid	Antibiotics	Lochner2012, Steneberg2007, Jarisch2004, **Sattler1990**			
Clonidine	Antihypertensive			**McGrath2009**	
Codeine	Analgesics				Lochner2012, Steneberg2007
Cyclophosphamide	Cytostatics	? **Tanaka2003**			
D-Cycloserine	Antibiotics	Steneberg2007, **Sattler1990**	Steneberg2007		
Diazepam	Tranquilizer	Lochner2012, Steneberg2007			
Diclofenac	NSAID				Lochner2012, Steneberg2007, Jarisch2004

Name	Detail	DAO inhibitors	Vitamin B6 antagonists	HNMT inhibitors	Mast cell degranulators
Dihydralazine	Antihypertensive	Lochner2012, Steneberg2007, **Wantke1998, Sattler1990**			
Diphenhydramine	Histamine H1-receptor antagonist			**Horton2005**	
Dobutamine	Antihypotonics	**Sattler1990**			
Flurbiprofen	NSAID				Lochner2012, Jarisch2004
Framycetin	Antibiotics	Steneberg2007			
Furosemide	Diuretics	Lochner2012, Steneberg2007			
Haloperidol	Antipsychotics	Lochner2012, Steneberg2007			
Heparin	Blood plasma replacement				Lochner2012
Hydroxychloroquine	Antimalarial			**Pacifici1992**	
Indometacin	NSAID				Lochner2012, Steneberg2007, Jarisch2004
Isoniazid	Antibiotics	Steneberg2007, Jarisch2004	Steneberg2007		
Ketoprofen	NSAID				Lochner2012, Steneberg2007, Jarisch2004
Meclofenamic acid	NSAID				Jarisch2004
Mefenamic acid	NSAID				Lochner2012, Steneberg2007, Jarisch2004
Metamizole	Analgesics	Lochner2012, Steneberg 2007, Jarisch 2004			
Metoclopramide	Drugs influencing gut motility	Lochner2012			
Metoprine	Antifolate			**Horton2005**	
Morphine	Analgesics				Lochner2012, Steneberg2007
Naproxen	NSAID				Lochner2012, Jarisch2004
Pancuronium	Muscle relaxants	Steneberg2007, **Sattler1990, Sattler1985**			Lochner2012
Pentamidine	Antibiotics	**Sattler1990**			
Pethidine	Analgesics				? Maintz2007
Polymyxin B	Antibiotics				Lochner2012
Prilocaine	Local analgesics				Lochner2012
Propafenone	Antiarrhythmics	Lochner2012, Jarisch2004			
Pyrimethamine	Antimalarial			**Pacifici1992**	
Quinidine	Antiarrhythmics	Steneberg2007			
Suxamethonium	Muscle relaxants				Lochner2012
Tacrine	Anticholinesterase			Horton2005	
Theophylline	Asthma drug	Lochner2012,			

Name	Detail	DAO inhibitors	Vitamin B6 antagonists	HNMT inhibitors	Mast cell degranulators
		Steneberg2007			
Thiopental	Narcotics				Lochner2012
D-Tubocurarine	Muscle relaxants	**Sattler1985**			Lochner2012, Steneberg2007
Vecuronium	Muscle relaxants			**Futo1988**	
Verapamil	Antihypertensive drugs	Lochner2012, Steneberg2007, Jarisch2004			

Table 14 Substances and food which inhibit enzymes

Substance	Food	HNMT	DAO	MAO unknown selectivity	MAO-A / MAO-B nonselective	MAO-A	MAO-B
phenylethylamine		Stratton1991	Stratton1991				
tyramine			Taylor-Lieber1979-rats	Stratton1991			
tryptamine			Stratton1991				
putrescine			Mongar1957-guinea pig ileum;				
cadaverine		Taylor-Lieber1979-rats	Mongar1957-guinea pig ileum; Taylor-Lieber1979-rats				
agmatine			Taylor-Lieber1979-rats				
anserine			Taylor-Lieber1979-rats				
carnosine			Taylor-Lieber1979-rats				
thiamine			Taylor-Lieber1979-rats				
nicotine		Gairola1988-guinea-pig					
tobacco smoke				yes			
Myristicin	Nutmeg, Parsley, Dill			wiki			
?	Liquorice			wiki			
?	Siberian Ginseng			wiki			
?	Yerba Mate			wiki			
?	Yohimbe			wiki			
Curcumin E100	Turmeric				wiki		
Anthocyanins E163					wiki		
Proanthocyanidin					wiki		
?	Ginkgo biloba				wiki		
?	Rhodiola rosea				wiki		
?	Ruta graveolens				wiki		
Harmala alkaloids	Coffee, Tobacco, Ayahuasca, Passion flower,					wiki	

Substance	Food	HNMT	DAO	MAO unknown selectivity	MAO-A / MAO-B nonselective	MAO-A	MAO-B
	Syrian rue, Tribulus terrestris						
Resveratrol	**Skin of red grapes**, Japanese knotweed					wiki	
Catechin	**Tea plant, Cocoa**, Cat's claw						wiki
Epicatechin	**Tea plant, Cocoa**, Cat's claw						wiki
Desmethoxyyangonin	Kava						wiki
Emodin	Fo-Ti						wiki
Hydroxytyrosol	**Olive oil**						wiki
Piperine	**Pepper**						wiki
?	Gentiana lutea						wiki

Table 15 Established fragrance contact allergens in humans

INCI name (or, if none exists, perfuming name according to CosIng)	Positive test reactions reported
acetylcedrene	+
amyl cinnamal	++
amyl cinnamyl alcohol	++
amyl salicylate	+
trans-anethole	+ (r.t.)
anisyl alcohol	+
benzaldehyde	+
benzyl alcohol	++
benzyl benzoate	++
benzyl cinnamate	++
benzyl salicylate	++
butylphenyl methylpropional (lilial®)	++
camphor	+ (r.t.)
beta-caryophyllene	Non-ox.: +, ox.: +
carvone	+ (r.t.)
cinnamal	+++
cinnamyl alcohol	+++
citral	+++
citronellol	++
coumarin	+++
(damascenone) rose ketone-4	+ (r.t.)
alpha-damascone (tmchb)	++
cis-beta-damascone	+
delta-damascone	+
dimethylbenzyl carbinyl acetate (dmbca)	+
eugenol	+++
farnesol	+++
geraniol	+++
hexadecanolactone	+ (r.t.)
hexamethylindanopyran	++
hexyl cinnamal	++
hydroxyisohexyl 3-cyclohexene carboxaldehyde (hicc)	++++
hydroxycitronellal	+++
isoeugenol	+++
alpha-isomethyl ionone	++
(dl)-limonene	++ (non-ox.); +++ (ox.)
linalool	++ (non-ox.); +++ (ox.)
linalyl acetate	+
menthol	++
6-methyl coumarin (photo-allergy)	++ (photo-allergy)
methyl 2-octynoate	++
methyl salicylate	+
3-methyl-5-(2,2,3-trimethyl-3-cyclopentenyl)pent-4-en-2-ol	++ (r.t.)
alpha-pinene and beta-pinene	++
propylidene phthalide	+ (r.t.)
salicylaldehyde	++

INCI name (or, if none exists, perfuming name according to CosIng)	Positive test reactions reported
alpha-santalol and beta-santalol	++
sclareol	+
terpineol (mixture of isomers)	+
alpha-terpineol	+
terpinolene	++
tetramethyl acetyloctahydronaphthalenes	+
trimethyl-benzenepropanol (majantol)	++
vanillin	++

Source: *Opinion on fragrance allergens in cosmetic products, European Commission 2012, SCCS/1459/11*

Legend:

"r.t." rarely tested. If a test allergen has been tested in less than 1,000 patients.

+ Up to 10 positive test reactions reported

++ 11 to 100

+++ 101 to 1000

++++ > 1000

Table 16 Natural extracts classified as established fragrance contact allergens in humans

INCI name (or, if none exists, $perfuming name according to CosIng)		Positive test reactions reported
cananga odorata and ylang-ylang oil	Cananga, Ylang-Ylang	+++
cedrus atlantica bark oil	Atlas Cedar bark	++
cinnamomum cassia leaf oil / cinnamomum zeylanicum bark oil	Cinnamon leaf / bark	++ (r.t.)
citrus aurantium amara flower / peel oil	Bitter orange flower / peel	++
citrus bergamia peel oil expressed$	Bergamot orange peel	+ (r.t.)
citrus limonum peel oil expressed	Sweet lemon peel	++
citrus sinensis (syn.: aurantium dulcis) peel oil expressed$	Orange peel	++
cymbopogon citratus / schoenanthus oils	Lemon grass / camel grass	++
eucalyptus spp. leaf oil$	Eucalyptus leaf	++
eugenia caryophyllus leaf / flower oil	Clove leaf / flower	+++
evernia furfuracea extract (tree moss)	Tree moss	+++
evernia prunastri extract (oak moss)	Oak moss	+++
jasminum grandiflorum / officinale	Spanish jasmine / Common jasmine	+++
juniperus virginiana	Eastern Juniper, Red Juniper	++
laurus nobilis	Bay laurel	++
lavandula hybrida	Lavender	+ (r.t.)
lavandula officinalis$	Common lavender	++
mentha piperita	Peppermint	++
mentha spicata	Spear Mint	++
myroxylon pereirae (balsam of peru)	**Peru Balsam**	++++
narcissus spp.	Narcissus, Daffodil	++
pelargonium graveolens	Geranium	++
pinus mugo/ pumila	Mountain Pine	++
pogostemon cablin	Siberian dwarf pine	++
rose flower oil (rosa spp.)	Rose flower	++
santalum album	Indian sandalwood	+++
turpentine (oil)	**Turpentine**	++++
verbena absolute	Verbena	++

Source: *Opinion on fragrance allergens in cosmetic products, European Commission 2012, SCCS/1459/11*
Legend:
"r.t." rarely tested. If a test allergen has been tested in less than 1,000 patients.
+ Up to 10 positive test reactions reported
++ 11 to 100
+++ 101 to 1000
++++ > 1000

Table 17 Shampoo ingredients

Shampoo	Body Shop, MINI RAINFOREST MOISTURE SHAMPOO, 5-1-2013	Body Shop, MINI RAINFOREST RADIANCE SHAMPOO, 5-1-2013	Body Shop, MINI RAINFOREST SHINE SHAMPOO, 5-1-2013	Dermolin Shampoo	Neutral, Shampoo, Alle haartypes, 0% parfum, 0% colorant, pH neutral	SebaMed, Shampoo alledag	Urtekram, No perfume shampoo Organic, 5-1-2013
Aqua (water)	+	+	+	+	+	+	+
Sucrose (sugar)	+	+	+				
Sodium Chloride (salt)	+	+	+	+	+		
Sodium Hydroxide	+	+	+				
Magnesium chloride				+			
Alcohol							+
Isopropyl Alcohol	+	+	+				
Phenoxyethanol						+	
Betaine				+			
Lauryl Betaine	+	+	+				
Cocamidopropyl betaine					+		+
Laureth-5 Carboxylic Acid	+	+	+				
PEG-18 glyceryl oleate/cocoate						+	
PEG-55 Propylene Glycol Oleate	+	+	+			+	
Glyceryl oleate							+
Caprylyl Glycol				+			
Propylene Glycol	+	+	+		+	+	
Hexylene Glycol					+		
Glycerin	+	+	+				+
Polyglyceryl-4 Caprate	+	+	+				
Glyceryl caprylate							+
Sucrose Laurate	+	+	+				
Polyquaternium-6	+	+	+				
Behenoyl PG-Trimonium chloride					+		
Hydroxypropyl oxidized starch PG-Trimonium chloride						+	
Coco-glucoside							+
Sodium coco-sulfate							+
Sodium laureth-sulfate				+	+		
Disodium laureth sulfosuccinate				+			
Sodium citrate						+	
Citric Acid	+	+	+		+		+
Tocopherol (vitamin E)	+	+	+				
Sodium cocoyl glutamate					+		+
Disodium Cocoyl glutamate	+	+	+				
Ethylhexyl Methoxycinnamate		+					
Lactic acid				+			

Shampoo	Body Shop, MINI RAINFOREST MOISTURE SHAMPOO, 5-1-2013	Body Shop, MINI RAINFOREST RADIANCE SHAMPOO, 5-1-2013	Body Shop, MINI RAINFOREST SHINE SHAMPOO, 5-1-2013	Dermolin Shampoo	Neutral, Shampoo, Alle haartypes, 0% parfum, 0% colorant, pH neutral	SebaMed, Shampoo alledag	Urtekram, No perfume shampoo Organic, 5-1-2013
Salicylic Acid	+	+	+				
Sorbic acid					+		
Disodium Lauroamphodiacetate				+			
C12-15 Alkyl lactate				+			
Piroctone olamine				+			
Polyo????-39				+			
Benzoic acid				+			
Decyl glucoside						+	
Sodium lauryl sulfoacetate						+	
Sodium Benzoate	+	+	+		+	+	
Geraniol			+				
Parfum	+	+	+			+	
Fragrance-free							+
Aloe Barbadensis Leaf Juice			+				
Camelina Sativa Seed Oil			+				
Linum Usitatissimum Seed Oil		+					
Mel (honey	+						
Olea Europaea Fruit Oil (Olive oil)			+				
Pentaclethra Macroloba Seed Oil	+	+	+				
Schinziophyton Rautanenii Kernel Oil	+						
Vaccinium Myrtillus Fruit Extract		+					
No paraben					+		
Danish Asthma and Allergy Association							+
Certified organic by Ecocert							+
No animal testing	+	+	+				+

Table 18 Toothpaste ingredients

Toothpaste	Elmex Sensitive	Parodontax Fluoride, actieve formule	Prodent, sterke tanden	Sensodyne, met fluoride
Aqua	+	+	+	+
Alcohol		+		
Alcohol denat.		+		
Hydrated silica	+		+	+
Silica dimethyl silylate	+			
Sodium bicarbonate		+		
Polyethylene	+			
Sodium phosphate			+	
Disodium phosphate			+	
Titanium dioxide	+			+
Cl 77891: titanium dioxide			+	
Sodium fluoride		+	+	+
Bis-(hydroxyethyl)amino-propyl-N-hydroxy-ethyl-octadecylamine-difluoride	+			
Olaflur	+			
Saccharin	+			
Sodium saccharin		+	+	+
Sorbitol	+		+	+
Propylene glycol			+	
PEG-6				+
Glycerin		+	+	+
Hydroxyethylcellulose	+			
Carrageenan			+	
Carbomer			+	
Cocamidopropyl betaine		+		+
Sodium C14-C16 olefin sulfonate			+	
Sodium lauryl sulfate				+
Potassium hydroxide	+			
Potassium nitrate				+
Xanthan Gum		+	+	+
Aroma	+		+	+
Echinacea Purpurea flower/leaf/stem juice		+		
Chamomilla Recutita extract		+		
Commiphora Myrrha Extract		+		
Krameria Triandra extract		+		
Mentha Arvensis oil		+		
Mentha Piperita oil		+		
Salvia Officinalis oil		+		
Limonene		+	+	+
Sodium benzoate		+		
Cl 77491 = iron oxide		+		
Cl 42051: blue			+	

Table 19 Fragrance allergens in food and flowers

Percentages: essential oil composition

Established contact allergens:	Cinnamal = Cinnamaldehyde	Cinnamyl Alcohol*	Citral	Coumarin	Eugenol*	Farnesol*	Geraniol*	Hydroxyisohexyl 3-cyclohexene carboxaldehyde	Isoeugenol*	Hydroxycitronellal	Limonene (oxidised)	Linalool* (oxidised)	Reference
SPICES:													
Bay leaf (Laurus nobilis)					+								
Black cumin (Nigella sativa) seeds											4,30%		5
Cinnamon (Cinnamomum verum)	90%	leaves		+	+							+	
Clove (Syzygium aromaticum)					72-90%								
Cardamom (Elletaria cardamomum)			0.36%				0.72%				2.4%	2.4%	2
Coriander (Coriandrum sativum) seeds							3.0%				5.0%	78.0%	2
Cumin (Cuminum cyminum) seeds													2
Ginger (Zinigiber officinale) rhizomes			0.7%								2.0%	0.6%	2
Juniper berry (Juniperus communis Linne. var erecta Pursch) fruit											20.00%	0.20%	2
Musterd seed (Brassica)													
Nutmeg (Myristica fragrans Houtt.) seeds					0.6%		0.4%		1.0%		7.0%	0.4%	2
Pepper, black (Piper nigrum)											23.0%	1.0%	2
Pepper, white											stripped	stripped	
Saffron (Crocus sativus)													
Turmeric with 5% curcumin (Curcuma longa)													
HERBS:													
Basil (Ocimum basilicum) flowering tops & leaves					0.5%						1.0%	1.1%	2
Chives													
Dill (Peucedanum graveolens)											45.0%	4.0%	2
Marjoram (Origanum majorana) leaves							0.3%				5.0%	25.0%	2
Peppermint (Mentha piperita)											3.0%	0.4%	2
Peppermint (Mentha arvensis L.)											3.0%	0.4%	1
Parsley (Petroselinum crispum)													
Rosemary (Rosemarinus officinalis) leaves & fresh flowering tops											6.0%	0.8%	2
Thyme (Thymus)												+	
TEA:													
Earl grey from peel of the bergamot orange			0.4%								40.0%	40.0%	1
Chamomile (Matricaria chamomilla recutica) flower											1.0%	0.4%	2
Jasmin (Jasminum officinale) flowers					1.80%	0.40%	0.10%					3.60%	2
Lemon myrtle (Backhousia citriodora)			90-98%										
Peppermint													
Rose flowers													

84

Established contact allergens:	Cinnamal = Cinnamaldehyde	Cinnamyl Alcohol*	Citral	Coumarin	Eugenol*	Farnesol*	Geraniol*	Hydroxyisohexyl 3-cyclohexene carboxaldehyde	Isoeugenol*	Hydroxycitronellal	Limonene (oxidised)	Linalool* (oxidised)	Reference
FLAVORS:													
Lemongrass (Cymbopogon nardus) -> Citronella oil			1.3%		1.0%	1.0%	25.0%				5.0%	1.5%	2
CITRUS FRUIT:													
Bergamot orange (Citrus bergamia) peel		0.4%									40.0%	40.0%	1
Bergamot orange (Citrus bergamia) peel unripe		0.7%									45.0%	15.0%	2
Grapefruit (Citrus grandis) peel		0.15%									95.0%	0.1%	2
Lemon (Citrus limonum) peel		3.0%					0.2%				73.0%	0.3%	1
Lemon (Citrus limonum) peel		3.0%					0.2%				73.0%	0.3%	2
Lime (Citrus aurantifolia, Rutaceae) fruit		3.0%					0.4%				50.0%	0.2%	2
Mandarin (Citrus nobilis) peel											92.0%	0.47%	2
Tangerine (Citrus reticulata) peel											95.0%	0.50%	2
Orange Sweet (Citrus sinensis) peel		0.1%									95.0%	0.4%	2
FRUIT:													
Apple													3
Avocado													
Banana													
Cherry													
Citrus fruit (see also above)							Geranial				+	+	3
Grape													
Mango											+		3
Papaya												+	3
Peach												+	3
Pear													
Pineapple		+					+				+	+	
Plum												+	3
Strawberry							+					+	3
WINE:													
* from oak barrel					+								4
Gewürztraminer							+					+	4
Riesling							+					+	4
Muscat							+					+	4
FLOWERS:													
Cyclamen						+							?
Geranium (Pelargonium graveolens) flowers		1.5%					18.0%				1.0%	8.5%	2
Geranium (Pelargonium graveolens P. roseum) flowers		1.5%					20.0%				1.0%	11.0%	2
Honeysuckle (Lonicera caprifolium and other Lonicera species) flowers		0.03%			0.4%	0.2%	1.5%				8.2%	1.7%	2
Hyacinth (Hyacinthus orientalis) flowers	0.017%	0.542%			0.021%	0.006%	0.006%		0.003%	0.400%	0.010%	3.331%	2
Lavender (Lavandula angustifolia P. Miller) flowers							1.1%				1.0%	45.0%	2
Narcissus													?

Established contact allergens:	Cinnamal = Cinnamaldehyde	Cinnamyl Alcohol*	Citral	Coumarin	Eugenol*	Farnesol*	Geraniol*	Hydroxyisohexyl 3-cyclohexene carboxaldehyde	Isoeugenol*	Hydroxycitronellal	Limonene (oxidised)	Linalool* (oxidised)	Reference

1: http://www.beebeautiful.org.uk/

2: http://www.essentialoilsdirect.co.uk/

3: Jiang YM, Song J. (2010) Fruits and Fruit Flavor: Classification and Biological Characterization, Chapter 1 in: Handbook of Fruit and Vegetable Flavors, John Wiley & Sons 2012

4: Robinson J (2006) The Oxford Companion to Wine, Oxford University Press, ISBN 978-0-19-860990-2, 813 pages

5: Nickavar B, Mojab F, Javidnia K, Amoli MA. (2003) Chemical Composition of the Fixed and Volatile Oils of Nigella sativa L. from Iran, Z Naturforsch C. 2003; 58(9-10): 629-31

Table 20 Acetaldehyde in food

	Number of samples	Acetaldehyde content (mg/kg)
Vegetables		
Cucumber	1	1.56
Carrot	1	1.91
Garlic	1	5.60
Cabbage turnip	1	2.88
Capsicum (yellow)	1	0.17
Capsicum (red)	1	0.10
Beetroot	1	0.15
Tomato	1	0.05
Onion	1	1.06
Pickled gherkin	1	2.61
Sweet corn (canned)	1	1.29
Sauerkraut (canned)	1	2.37
Asparagus (canned)	1	0.40
Carrots (canned)	1	1.60
Peas (canned)	1	4.49
Fresh beans (canned)	2	1.01
Lentils (canned)	1	0.10
Other foods		
Strawberry jam	1	0.26
Plum puree	1	0.97
Honey	1	1.01
Wheat and rye bread	1	1.50
Rye whole-meal bread with pumpkinseed	1	2.68
Vinegar	1	2.61
Mustard	1	0.15
Lemon flavour for baking	1	**26.32**
Orange flavour	1	**1416.00**
Alcohol-free beverages		
Pineapple juice (direct juice)	1	0.01
Apple juice (direct juice)	1	5.72
Banana nectar	2	0.26-0.45
Peach nectar	1	0.52
Orange juice (from concentrate)	1	1.83
Orange juice (direct juice)	1	5.89
Smoothie strawberry banana	1	3.06
Grape juice (direct juice)	1	0.97
Ice tea (peach flavour)	1	4.32
Energy drink	3	0.06-1.08
Soft drink (with fermented cranberry)	1	3.49
Soft drink (with fermented quince)	1	0.32
Soft drink (with fermented herbs)	1	0.33
Cola	1	0.28
Apple soft drink	1	7.54
Cherry soft drink	1	0.93
Orange soft drink	2	**14.01-16.30**
Wild beery soft drink	1	2.39
Carrot juice (fermented)	1	1.19

	Number of samples	Acetaldehyde content (mg/kg)
Carrot juice (direct juice)	1	2.49
Tomato juice (from concentrate)	1	0.15
Instant coffee (powder)	2	**31.20-35.51**
Instant coffee A (2 g per 180mL)	1	0.26
Coffee, roasted (powder)	3	1.15-**40.14**
Earl Grey tea (leaves) (powder)	1	9.84
Green tea (leaves) (powder)	1	1.35

Source: Uebelacker 2011

Table 21 Lipids in food

High content of polyunsaturated fatty acids means high risk to develop rancidity.

Name	Description	Total poly-unsaturated fatty acids	Total mono-unsaturated fatty acids	Total saturated fatty acids
NUTS				
Walnut	Nuts, walnuts, english	**47.2%**	8.9%	6.1%
Pine nuts	Nuts, pine nuts, dried	**34.1%**	18.8%	4.9%
Pecannut	Nuts, pecans	**21.6%**	40.8%	6.2%
Brazil nut	Nuts, brazilnuts, dried, unblanched	**20.6%**	24.5%	15.1%
Peanut	Peanuts, all types, raw	15.6%	24.4%	6.8%
Pistachio	Nuts, pistachio nuts, raw	13.7%	23.8%	5.6%
Almond	Nuts, almonds	12.1%	30.9%	3.7%
Hazelnut	Nuts, hazelnuts or filberts	7.9%	45.7%	4.5%
Cashewnut	Nuts, cashew nuts, raw	7.8%	23.8%	7.8%
Macadamia nuts	Nuts, macadamia nuts, raw	1.5%	58.9%	12.1%
Chestnut	Nuts, chestnuts, european, raw, peeled	0.5%	0.4%	0.2%
Coconut	Nuts, coconut meat, raw	0.4%	1.4%	29.7%
SEEDS				
Poppy Seed	Spices, poppy seed	**28.6%**	6.0%	4.5%
Chia Seeds	Seeds, chia seeds, dried	**23.7%**	2.3%	3.3%
Sunflower Seeds	Seeds, sunflower seed kernels, dried	**23.1%**	18.5%	4.5%
Sesame Seeds	Seeds, sesame seeds, whole, dried	**21.8%**	18.8%	7.0%
Pumpkin Seeds	Seeds, pumpkin and squash seed kernels, dried	**21.0%**	16.2%	8.7%
OIL				
Flaxseed Oil	Oil, flaxseed, cold pressed	**67.8%**	18.4%	9.0%
Sunflower Oil	Oil, sunflower, linoleic, (approx. 65%)	**65.7%**	19.5%	10.3%
Sesame Seed Oil	Oil, sesame, salad or cooking	**41.7%**	39.7%	14.2%
Sunflower Oil	Oil, sunflower, linoleic (less than 60%)	**40.1%**	45.4%	10.1%
Sunflower Oil	Oil, sunflower, linoleic, (partially hydrogenated)	**36.4%**	46.2%	13.0%
Canola (Rapeseed) Oil	Oil, canola	**28.1%**	63.3%	7.4%
Olive Oil	Oil, olive, salad or cooking	10.5%	73.0%	13.8%
Sunflower Oil	Oil, sunflower, high oleic (70% and over)	3.8%	83.7%	9.9%
Coconut Oil	Oil, coconut	1.8%	5.8%	86.5%
GRAINS				
Quinoa	Quinoa, uncooked	3.3%	1.6%	0.7%
Maize/Corn	Corn, yellow	2.2%	1.3%	0.7%
Spelt	Spelt, uncooked	1.3%	0.4%	0.4%
Rye	Rye	0.8%	0.2%	0.2%
Rice	Rice, brown, long-grain, cooked	0.3%	0.3%	0.2%
Rice	Rice, brown, medium-grain, cooked	0.3%	0.3%	0.2%
CEREALS				
Oats	Cereals, oats, regular and quick, not fortified, dry	2.3%	2.0%	1.1%
Maize/Corn	Cereals ready-to-eat, KELLOGG, KELLOGG'S Corn Flakes	0.2%	0.1%	0.1%
FLOUR				

Name	Description	Total poly-unsaturated fatty acids	Total mono-unsaturated fatty acids	Total saturated fatty acids
Oats	Oat flour, partially debranned	3.3%	2.9%	1.6%
Millet	Millet flour	2.6%	0.9%	0.5%
Corn	Corn flour, whole-grain, yellow	1.8%	1.0%	0.5%
Sorghum flour	Sorghum flour	1.4%	0.9%	0.5%
Wheat	Wheat flour, whole-grain	1.2%	0.3%	0.4%
Rye	Rye flour, dark	1.0%	0.3%	0.3%
Rice	Rice flour, brown	1.0%	1.0%	0.6%
Buckwheat	Buckwheat flour, whole-groat	0.9%	0.9%	0.7%
Triticale	Triticale flour, whole-grain	0.8%	0.2%	0.3%
Barley	Barley flour or meal	0.8%	0.2%	0.3%
CHOCOLATE				
Chocolate, dark	Chocolate, dark, 45- 59% cacao solids	1.1%	9.5%	18.5%
Chocolate, dark	Chocolate, dark, 60-69% cacao solids	1.2%	11.5%	22.0%
Chocolate, dark	Chocolate, dark, 70-85% cacao solids	1.3%	12.8%	24.5%
DAIRY				
Milk	Milk, fluid, 1% fat, without added vitamin A and vitamin D	0.0%	0.3%	0.6%
Milk, non-fat	Milk, nonfat, fluid, without added vitamin A and vitamin D (fat free or skim)	0.0%	0.0%	0.1%
Buttermilk	Milk, buttermilk, fluid, whole	0.2%	0.8%	1.9%
Yogurt, whole milk	Yogurt, plain, whole milk, 8 grams protein per 8 ounce	0.1%	0.9%	2.1%
Yogurt, low fat	Yogurt, plain, low fat, 12 grams protein per 8 ounce	0.0%	0.4%	1.0%
Yogurt, Greek, plain, nonfat	Yogurt, Greek, plain, nonfat	0.0%	0.1%	0.1%
Cheese, brie	Cheese, brie	0.8%	8.0%	17.4%
Cheese, camembert	Cheese, camembert	0.7%	7.0%	15.3%
Cheese, cheddar	Cheese, cheddar	0.9%	9.4%	21.1%
Cheese, edam	Cheese, edam	0.7%	8.1%	17.6%
Cheese, feta	Cheese, feta	0.6%	4.6%	14.9%
Cheese, gouda	Cheese, gouda	0.7%	7.7%	17.6%
Cheese, mozzarella	Cheese, mozzarella, whole milk	0.8%	6.6%	13.2%
...				
MEAT				
Bacon (pork)	Pork, cured, bacon, cooked, baked	4.9%	19.1%	14.2%
Chicken breast	Chicken breast tenders, cooked, conventional oven	3.0%	6.8%	3.8%
Chicken wing	Chicken, broilers or fryers, wing, meat and skin, cooked, stewed	3.6%	6.6%	4.7%

Source:
United States Department of Agriculture, National Nutrient Database for Standard Reference, Release 25 (Access date 2 January 2013)
http://ndb.nal.usda.gov/ ndb/search/list

Table 22 Benzoates in food

Benzoates are used as food preservative.

<u>E-numbers:</u>

E209   Heptyl p-hydroxybenzoate
E210   Benzoic acid
E211   Sodium benzoate
E212   Potassium benzoate
E213   Calcium benzoate
E214   Ethylparaben (ethyl para-hydroxybenzoate)
E215   Sodium ethyl para-hydroxybenzoate
E216   Propylparaben (propyl para-hydroxybenzoate)
E217   Sodium propyl para-hydroxybenzoate
E218   Methylparaben (methyl para-hydroxybenzoate)
E219   Sodium methyl para-hydroxybenzoate

Naturally occurring benzoic acid in foods:
- **Cinnamon**
- **Ripe cloves**
- **Cranberries**
- **Prunes**
- **Greengage plums**
- **Apples**

Source: http://en.wikipedia.org/wiki/Sodium_benzoate

The spices cinnamon and cloves are used in:
- **Ontbijtkoek** (Dutch), **kruidkoek** (Belgian)
- **Speculaas** (Dutch)
- **Pepernoten** (Dutch), **kruidnoten** (Belgian)
- **Koekkruiden** (Dutch), **speculaaskruiden** (Belgian): a mixture of cinnamon, nutmeg, clove, ginger, cardamom en white pepper
- **Mulled wine**, **Glühwein** (German). It is usually prepared from red wine, heated and spiced with cinnamon sticks, vanilla pods, cloves, star aniseed, citrus, and sugar (http://en.wikipedia.org/wiki/Mulled_wine).

Table 23 Nitrites and Nitrates in food

Nitrates are used as a **food preservative**.

<u>E-numbers:</u>
E249: KNO2 potassium nitrite
E250: NaNO2 sodium nitrite
E251: NaNO3 sodium nitrate
E252: KNO3 potassium nitrate

The European Commission has set rules for *organic* production, labelling and control (European Commission 2008). For meat products:
- E 250: indicative ingoing amount expressed as NaNO2: 80 mg/kg
- E 250: maximum residual amount expressed as NaNO2: 50 mg/kg
- E 252: indicative ingoing amount expressed as NaNO3: 80 mg/kg
- E 252: maximum residual amount expressed as NaNO3: 50 mg/kg

"This additive can only be used, if it has been demonstrated to the satisfaction of the competent authority that no technological alternative, giving the same guarantees and/or allowing to maintain the specific features of the product, is available."

Nitrate rich vegetables

Table 4. Classification of vegetables according to NO_3 content (mg kg^{-1} fm)

Very low (<200)	Low (200–500)	Middle (500–1000)	High (1000–2500)	Very high (>2500)
Artichoke	Broccoli	Cabbage	Celeriac	Celery
Asparagus	Carrot	'Cima di rapa' (broccoli rab)	Chinese cabbage	Chervil
Broad bean	Cauliflower	Dill	Endive	Cress
Brussels sprouts Eggplant	Cucumber	'Radicchio'	Escarola	Lamb's lettuce
Garlic	Pumpkin	Savoy cabbage	Fennel	Lettuce
Onion	'Puntarelle' chicory	Turnip	Kohlrabi	Radish
Green bean			Leaf chicory	Red beetroot
Melon			Leek	Rocket
Mushroom			Parsley	Spinach
Pea				Swiss chard
Pepper				
Potato				
Summer squash				
Sweet potato				
Tomato				
Watermelon				

Source: Santamaria 2006

Table 24 Sulfites and related compounds in food

Sulfites are used as a food preservative.

E-numbers:
E220 Sulphur dioxide
E221 Sodium sulphite
E222 Sodium bisulphite (sodium hydrogen sulphite)
E223 Sodium metabisulphite
E224 Potassium metabisulphite
E225 Potassium sulphite
E226 Calcium sulphite
E227 Calcium hydrogen sulphite (also firming agent)
E228 Potassium hydrogen sulphite
Legal limits for *labeling*:
- US: >10 mg/kg or mg/liter expressed as SO2
- EU: >10 mg/kg or mg/liter expressed as SO2 (DIRECTIVE 2000/13/EC)

Legal limits for *content*:
- EU: < 160 mg/liter in red wine (sugar < 5 g/liter)
- EU: < 210 mg/liter in red wine (sugar > 5 g/liter)
- EU: < 210 mg/liter in white & rosé wine (sugar < 5 g/liter)
- EU: < 260 mg/liter in white & rosé wine (sugar > 5 g/liter)

Wine
- Sulfites occur naturally in all wines to some extent. Organic wines are not necessarily sulfite-free.
- Sulfites are commonly introduced to arrest fermentation at a desired time, and may also be added to wine as preservatives to prevent spoilage and oxidation at several stages of the winemaking.
- Sulfur dioxide protects wine from not only oxidation, but also bacteria.
- Without sulfites, grape juice would turn to vinegar.
- In general, sweet (dessert) wines contain more sulfites than dry wines, and some sweet white wines contain more sulfites than red wines.
- Store your wine < 15°C.

Other foods:
- **Dried fruits** (for example raisins, dates, prunes, figs, apricots, peaches, apples and pears)
- **Preserved radish**
- **Dried potato products** (for example chips)
- **Shrimp** are sometimes treated with sulfites on fishing vessels

Source: http://en.wikipedia.org/wiki/Sulfite

Table 25 Histidine and estimated theoretical maximum concentrations of histamine in food

Food high in histidine has the *potential* to develop high levels of histamine.

Food	Description	Histidine	Histamine CALCULATED THEORETICAL MAXIMUM
		g per 100 g	mg per kg
FISH			
Anchovy	Fish, anchovy, european, raw	0.599	4291
Cod	Fish, cod, Atlantic, raw	0.524	3754
Haddock	Fish, haddock, raw	0.557	3990
Herring	Fish, herring, Atlantic, raw	0.529	3790
Mackerel	Fish, mackerel, Atlantic, raw	0.548	3926
Salmon			
Sardine			
Trout			
Tuna	**Fish, tuna, fresh, bluefin, raw**	**0.687**	4922
Tuna	**Fish, tuna, fresh, skipjack, raw**	**0.648**	4642
Tuna	**Fish, tuna, fresh, yellowfin, raw**	**0.688**	4929
CRUSTACEANS			
Crab	Crustaceans, crab, alaska king, raw	0.372	2665
Crab	Crustaceans, crab, blue, raw	0.367	2629
Crab	Crustaceans, crab, dungeness, raw	0.354	2536
Crab	Crustaceans, crab, queen, raw	0.376	2694
Shrimp	Crustaceans, shrimp, mixed species, raw	0.300	2149
MOLLUSK			
Mussel	Mollusks, mussel, blue, raw	0.228	1633
Oyster	Mollusks, oyster, eastern, farmed, raw	0.100	716
Oyster	Mollusk, oyster, eastern, wild, raw	0.110	788
Oyster	Mollusk, oyster, eastern, Pacific, raw	0.181	1297
MEAT			
Chicken	Chicken, broilers or fryers, breast, meat only, raw	0.791	5667
Pork	Pork, fresh, leg (ham), whole, separable lean and fat, raw	0.659	4721
BEANS			
Lentils	Lentils, raw	0.727	5208
Peas	Peas, green, raw	0.107	767
Soy bean	Soy beans, green, raw	0.348	2493

NUTS			
Almond	Nuts, almonds	0.557	3990
Brazil nut	Nuts, brazilnuts, dried, unblanched	0.386	2765
Cashewnut	Nuts, cashew nuts, raw	0.456	3267
Chestnut	Nuts, chestnuts, european, raw, peeled	0.045	322
Coconut	Nuts, coconut meat, raw	0.077	552
Hazelnut			
Macadamia nuts			
Peanut	Peanuts, all types, raw	0.652	4671
Pecannut	Nuts, pecans	0.262	1877
Pine nuts	Nuts, pine nuts, dried	0.341	2443
Pistachio	Nuts, pistachio nuts, raw	0.503	3604
Pistachio	Nuts, pistachio nuts, dry roasted, without salt added	0.513	3675
Walnut	Nuts, walnuts, english	0.391	2801
GRAINS			
Barley	Barley flour or meal	0.236	1691
Buckwheat	Buckwheat flour, whole-groat	0.294	2106
Corn			
Millet	Millet flour	0.257	1841
Oats	Oats	0.405	2901
Rice	Rice, brown, long-grain, raw	0.202	1447
Rice	Rice, brown, medium-grain, raw	0.190	1361
Rye	Rye	0.189	1354
Rye	Rye flour, dark	0.233	1669
Rye	Rye flour, medium	0.159	1139
Rye	Rye flour, light	0.147	1053
Sorghum	Sorghum	0.246	1762
Sorghum	Sorghum flour	0.156	1118
Triticale	Triticale	0.311	2228
Triticale	Triticale flour, whole-grain	0.314	2250
Wheat	Wheat flour, whole-grain	0.357	2558
VEGETABLES			
Eggplant	Eggplant, raw	0.023	165
Tomato	Tomato, red, ripe, raw, year round average	0.014	100
White cabbage	Cabbage, raw	0.022	158

	molecular weight	molecular weight
	155.15	111.15

USDA Food Composition Database
Software: USDA Food Search for Windows, version 1.0, database version SR25, downloaded 15 January 2013
http://www.ars.usda.gov/Services/docs.htm?docid=5720

Table 26 Sum of biogenic amines in food samples with available concentrations of histamine, tyramine, putrescine and cadaverine

Source: EFSA 2011, p. 42

Food class	Sub-category	n	Histamine Mean (mg/kg)	Histamine P95 (mg/kg)	Tyramine Mean (mg/kg)	Tyramine P95 (mg/kg)	Putrescine Mean (mg/kg)	Putrescine P95 (mg/kg)	Cadaverine Mean (mg/kg)	Cadaverine P95 (mg/kg)	Sum of BAs Mean (mg/kg)	Sum of BAs P95 (mg/kg)
Alcoholic beverages	Beer	188	1.4	4.8	6.1	24.7	3.3 - 3.5	8.3	1.3 - 1.5	5.3	12.1 - 12.4	36.7
	Fortified and liqueur wines	28	1.1	2.8	6	21.3	1.4	3.6	0.1	0.3	8.6	26.4
	Wine, white, sparkling	45	1	5.2	4.9	26.4	5.2	15	<0.1	0.2	11.1	46.1
Condiment	Fish sauce	71	198 - 199	597	105 - 107	421	98.1 - 99	167	180 - 182	502	582 - 588	1500
	Other savoury sauces	27	0.5 - 10.1	<13.3	1.5 - 10	18.6	6 - 13.6	24.2	3 - 12.7	<17	11 - 47	24.2 - 56
Fish and fish products	Fermented Fish products	68	7.7 - 11.4	31.5	45.5 - 47	136	12.2 - 15	75.1	14.4 - 17	34.5	79.8 - 91	552 - 572
Meat products	Fermented sausages	369	23.2 - 23	149	136	397	84.2 - 84	334	37.4 - 38	154	281 - 283	889
	Other ripened meat products	92	6 - 6.2	35	44 - 44.2	149	32.8	136	17.2 - 17	84.1	100 - 101	342
	Other meat products	75	3.9 - 4.4	4.8	16.1 - 16	67	17.4 - 17	123	6.7 - 6.8	25	44 - 45	151
Dairy products	Cheese	2136	20.6 - 61	127	59 - 98	420	25.4 - 65	143	72.2 - 109	472	177 - 334	1050
	Fresh cheese	98	3.2 - 38	20 - 50	12.8 - 48	89	5.5 - 41	4 - 50	10.7 - 45	33.8 - 50	32.1 - 172	323 - 464
	Hard cheese	1062	25 - 65	136	67.1 - 103	475	26.6 - 65	132	47.8 - 83	235	167 - 318	940 - 1030
	Washed rind cheese	676	8.5 - 54	46 - 50	31.6 - 76	240	32.3 - 72	182	147 - 186	989	220 - 388	1420 - 1516
	Blue cheese	296	21.3 - 63	149	63.2 - 10	453	20.9 - 62	149	83.1 - 12	519	188 - 351	1100 - 1184
	Acid curd cheese	4	51.3 - 55	102	335	480	449	648	628	980	1460	2140
	Yoghurt	7	0.5	1	1.9	5.2	0.7	1.1	3.2	10.3	6.3	12
	Other dairy products	4	0.3	0.6	0.3	0.4	0.7	0.9	1.9	3	3.1	4.8
Vegetables and vegetable products	Fermented vegetables	9	39.4 - 42	92	45 - 47.4	91	264	549	26 - 35.4	94	375 - 390	747
	Other vegetables	14	5.4	75.7	1.8	25.4	37.2	310	17	85	61.4	422

The statistics are presented using a bounded approach for the handling of non-detected/non-quantified data (therefore they are displayed as ranges). The upper bound of the range estimates the non-detected/non-quantified values using the reported limit of detection (LOD) or limit of quantification (LOQ) respectively. The lower bound of the range instead assumes the non-detected/non-quantified values as zero. When the lower bound and the upper bound of the range are coincident, only one number is presented. When the lower bound is zero, the range is represented by the upper bound prefixed by '<'. The table contains the number of samples (n), the mean and the 95-percentile (P95).

Table 27 Biogenic amine concentrations in food

Concentrations in mg/kg.

No	Name	Detail	Histamine	Phenyl-ethylamine	Tyramine	Tryptamine	Serotonine	Ethylamine
			mg/kg	mg/kg	mg/kg	mg/kg	mg/kg	mg/kg
65	DAIRY							
66	Año, Spanish cheese		113					
67	Azeitão, Portuguese sheep cheese, raw milk		644-682		358-445			
68	Blue cheeses		6.6 (0-376.6)		14.4 (0-1585.4)	3.2 (0-128.8)		
70	Blue vein cheese, pasteurized milk	7 weeks ripening	<DL-90	<DL	10-185	<DL-6		
71	Blue-veined cheese		13.9 (0.8-20.2)		32.0 (8.3-58.4)	3.6 (2.1-5.4)		
72	Brie cheese		2		440			
73	Brie cheese from farmhouse		87		932			
74	Camembert cheese		5		154	60		
75	Camembert cheese from farmhouse		250		821			
77	Castelmagno		645.8		1009.1	1048.7		
78	Cheddar cheese		1710	40	783	1		
79	Cheddar cheese	Egypt	13		22			
82	Cheddar cheese, ripened							
83	Cheddar cheese, young							
84	Cottage cheese		0	()	1.3			
86	Danish blue (Danablu) cheese		341		700			
87	Dutch cheese		52.0 (0-350.0)		138.0 (0-625.0)			
88	Dutch-type cheese, hard, pasteurized milk	22 weeks ripening	2-17	1-54	16-300	1-2		
89	Dutch-type cheese, semihard, pasteurized milk	25 weeks ripening	22-59		5-392			
90	Edam cheese, young		3	12	141			
91	Egyptian blue cheese				2010			
92	Emmentaler cheese		283		437			

No	Name	Detail	Histamine	Phenyl-ethylamine	Tyramine	Tryptamine	Serotonine	Ethylamine
93	Feta cheese		14		560			
94	Feta cheese, Greek goat/sheep, brined, thermized milk	17 weeks ripening	85	5	246	6		
95	Goat cheese		33		791			
96	Goat cheese	13 weeks ripening	10	37	68	22		
97	Goat cheese, raw milk	13 weeks ripening	43-83	27-92	325-428	12		
98	Goat cheeses		1.3 (0-88.4)		8.5 (0-830.5)	0.6 (0-17.4)		
99	Gorgonzola cheese		1275		1255			
100	Gouda cheese		350	46	625	(200)		
101	Gouda cheese	Egypt	8		10			
102	Gouda cheese	12 weeks ripening	178-418		337-776			
103	Grana Padano cheese	Italy	11-430		7-87			
104	Grana type cheese	Italy	74-647		6-254			
105	Gruyère cheese		20		88			
106	Hard-ripened cheese from pasteurized milk		4.0 (0-163.6)		7.2 (0-301.4)	0.9 (0-45.1)		
107	Hard-ripened cheese from raw milk		18.3 (0-391.4)		125.5 (0-609.4)	0.3 (0-33.8)		
108	Maasdam cheese		246		417			
109	Manchego, Spanish cheese		109					
110	Mascarpone		527	23	1521			
113	Mozzarella		0		6			
114	Parmesan cheese		277		75			
115	Parmesan cheese		152					
116	Parmigiano Reggiano cheese		85-679		5-80			
117	Pecorino di Farindola cheese	90 days ripening, Italy, 10 farms	0-22	0-127	52-1171			13-482
118	Processed cheese		<DL	8-400	4-160	<DL		
119	Processed cheese		1	1-2	1-29	1		
120	Raclette cheese		1					
121	Ras, Egyptian cheese	Egypt	17		15			
122	Raschera		452.4		153.9	389.9		
123	Roquefort cheese		64	71	548	(1100)		

No	Name	Detail	Histamine	Phenyl-ethylamine	Tyramine	Tryptamine	Serotonine	Ethylamine
124	Semihard Italian cheese, unpasteurized milk	21 weeks ripening	117-378	8-20	128-394	2-5		
125	Semisoft cheese, pasteurized milk	20 weeks ripening	<DL-124	5-179	39-770			
126	Semisoft cheese, raw milk	20 weeks ripening	226-573	29-223	400-1478			
127	Sheep cheese		64		145			
128	Sheep cheese, Portuguese, traditional, raw milk	9 weeks ripening	16	9	176	56		
129	Spanish retail cheeses, ripened		2-164	<DL-29	<DL-242	<DL-45		
130	Spanish retail cheeses, unripened		<DL	<DL	<1	<DL		
131	Spanish traditional cheeses		<DL-928		10-1807			
132	Spreadable cheese, Dutch		0		50			
133	Spreadable cheese, non-Dutch		76	60	164	4		
134	Swiss cheese		500		100			
135	Swiss-type cheese	24 weeks ripening	750-1290		64-910			
136	Tilsiter cheese		184		510			
137	Toma piemontese		587.6		282.3	255.5		
138	Unripened cheese		0		0 (0-0.6)	0		
140	Yogurt		<1		<1			
141	SEAFOOD & PRODUCTS							
142	Anchovy paste		3440	75	64			
143	Anchovy sauce		216					
144	Anchovy, canned		952	50	130	90		
145	Anchovy, canned	Taiwan	32 (0-75)		1 (0-2)	8 (0-16)		
146	Anchovy, fresh, summer	Taiwan	14-136					
147	Anchovy, fresh, winter	Taiwan	41-83					
148	Anchovy, salt ripened		9.8 (4.5-19.4)		71.5 (40.2-89.5)			
149	Bloater (herring)		75		29			
150	Bonito, canned	Taiwan	14 (0-35)		3 (0-5)	0		
151	Cod		1		0			
152	Crab		0		0			

No	Name	Detail	Histamine	Phenyl-ethylamine	Tyramine	Tryptamine	Serotonine	Ethylamine
154	Eel, fresh and fumed		0		0			
156	Fish meal, dried		273					
157	Fish paste		263 (101-760)	0	9 (0-32)			
158	Fish sauce		394 (45-1220)	4 (0-42)	9 (0-42)			
159	Fish sauce, from Far East		0-729	0-251	0-1178			
160	Fish, canned		5					
161	Haddock liver		60		20			
162	Haddock, fresh and frozen		0		0			
163	Haddock, fumed		0		0			
164	Hake, fresh		<1		<1			
165	Herring, in tomato sauce		8	0	0			
166	Herring, pickled		(3500)		(3030)			
167	Herring, salted		29		19			
168	Herring, vinegar		8	14	2			
169	Mackerel, canned		14	2	7			
170	Mackerel, canned	Taiwan	11 (0-24)		0	2 (0-6)		
171	Mackerel, fresh		46	0	0			
172	Mackerel, fresh, summer	Taiwan	10-44					
173	Mackerel, fresh, winter	Taiwan	11-25					
174	Mackerel, fumed		127	17	25			
175	Mackerel, salted, retail market	Northern Taiwan	3.4 (0-14.1)		0	0		
176	Mackerel, salted, retail market	Southern Taiwan	26.0 (0-120.2)		0	0		
177	Mackerel, salted, supermarket	Northern Taiwan	4.5 (0-15.0)		0	0		
178	Mackerel, salted, supermarket	Southern Taiwan	21.4 (0-70.1)		0	0		
179	Marlin, fresh, summer	Taiwan	4-125					
180	Marlin, fresh, winter	Taiwan	4-24					
181	Milk fish, canned	Taiwan	2 (0-5)		0	0		
182	Mussels: fresh, vinegar and canned		0		0			
184	Pacific saury, canned	Taiwan	12 (0-12)		2 (0-5)	0		
185	Plaice, fresh and baked		1		0			
186	Pollock		0		0			
188	Salmon,		7		0			

No	Name	Detail	Histamine	Phenyl-ethylamine	Tyramine	Tryptamine	Serotonine	Ethylamine
	canned							
189	Salmon, fresh		1		10			
191	Salmon, smoked		149		129			
192	Sardines, canned		164		0			
195	Shrimp paste		382 (20-1180)	30 (0-91)	4 (0-19)			
196	Shrimps		2	0	28			
197	Sprat, canned		0		0			
198	Tarasi (shrimp paste)		100	446	1780	9		
199	Trout rainbow, fresh		0		0			
200	Trout, smoked		0		0			
201	Tub Gurnard / Tom Grimard		30					
202	Tuna, canned		22	45	37			
203	Tuna, canned	Taiwan	45 (0-187)		2 (0-4)	2 (0-3)		
204	Tuna, fresh		98		0			
205	Tuna, fresh, red muscle		2.0		0.5			
206	Tuna, fresh, white muscle		6.2		1.6			
208	Whiting		0		0			
209	MEAT & EGG							
210	Alheira, Portugese smoked fermented sausage		0.1-3.0	0-77.5	0.7-63.2			0-21.1
212	Bovine meat				10.7	20.4		
213	Chicken liver		7		51			
214	Chicken meat		9	0	22			
216	Cow liver		1		4			
217	Cow meat		1		31			
218	Cow meat, chopped		7		40			
219	Deli sandwich (cooked product of meat and salmon)	Spain	0.5		1			
223	Ham meat, cooked		8	14	78	22		
224	Ham, cooked		0 (0-0.9)		1.0 (0-78.0)			
225	Ham, cooked with fibre (Bioyork)	Spain	<DL		6			
226	Ham, cooked, sliced, high pressure	Spain	0.3		4			
227	Ham, cooked, sliced, protective atmophere packed	Spain	0.2		2			
228	Ham, cooked, sliced, vacuum packed	Spain	0.2		32			

No	Name	Detail	Histamine	Phenyl-ethylamine	Tyramine	Tryptamine	Serotonine	Ethylamine
229	Ham, cured, sliced, protective atmosphere packed	Spain	2		6			
230	Ham, cured, sliced, vacuum packed	Spain	2		5			
231	Ham, dry-cured, Italian	15 months old	0		40.2 (0-110)			
232	Ham, dry-cured, Italian	23 months old	0		72.4 (1.0-274)			
233	Ham, dry-cured, Spanish		0.8 (0-150.0)		0.7 (0-46.5)			
234	Ham, raw		271	51	254	67		
235	Hare liver		31	0	560			
236	Hare meat		50	0	21			
239	Liver sausage		0		0			
241	Loin, pickled, non-packed	Spain	1		11			
242	Loin, pickled, protective atmosphere packed	Spain	2		9			
243	Loin, steak, non-packed	Spain	0.2		7			
244	Loin, steak, protective atmosphere packed	Spain	0.3		12			
245	Meat extract, dry		8	0	231			
246	Mortadella, Spanish		0 (0-4.8)		2.5 (0-67.0)			
247	Poličane		28.5 (25-32)		89 (86-92)	5 (5-5)		
248	Pork meat		5	14	25	29		
249	Pork meat chopped		8		39			
253	Sausage, dry (various)		63	50	310	31		
254	Sausage, Dutch, dry, Rotterdammer		70	8	95			
255	Sausage, ripened fermented	France	0-42	0-54	5-227	0-19		
256	Sausage, ripened fermented	Greece	0-106	0-21	12-272	0-48		
257	Sausage, ripened fermented	Italy	0-9	0-43	60-303	0-17		
258	Sausage, ripened fermented	Portugal	0-95	0-46	9-269	0-36		
259	Sausage, ripened fermented	Slovakia	0-15	0-5	0-118	0-2		
260	Sausage,	Spain	0-133	0-31	38-474	0-79		

No	Name	Detail	Histamine	Phenyl-ethylamine	Tyramine	Tryptamine	Serotonine	Ethylamine
	ripened fermented							
261	Sausages, Belgian		4.1 (0-19.7)		36.8 (10.2-150.6)			
262	Sausages, Belgian North		1		76	17		
263	Sausages, Belgian South		18		176	39		
264	Sausages, Danish		9 (1-56)		54 (5-110)	27 (0-91)		
265	Sausages, Egyptian		5.3 (7.5-41)		14 (9.5-53)	13 (2.5-34)		
266	Sausages, fermented		11 (1-3)?		110 (40-10)?			
267	Sausages, Finnish		54 (0-180)		88 (4-200)	14 (0-43)		
268	Sausages, French saucisson, industrial		71 (16-151)		220 (172-268)	3.9 (0-9)		
269	Sausages, French saucisson, traditional		15.3 (15-16)		164.3 (84-217)			
270	Sausages, German Mettwurst		21 (0-170)		72 (5-320)	18 (0-54)		
271	Sausages, Italian		0		187	19		
272	Sausages, Italian salsiccia		0		76.7 (0-338.9)			
273	Sausages, Italian, Salami, Soppressata	Italy	21.9 (0-100.9)		178 (0-556.9)			
274	Sausages, Italian, Salamini italiani alla cacciatora PDO	Italy	165		372			
275	Sausages, Norwegian		1		12	9		
276	Sausages, Portugese Painho de Portalegre, 3% NaCl		0		356.5	3.2		
277	Sausages, Portugese Painho de Portalegre, 6% NaCl		0		257.4	0		
278	Sausages, Russian		89 (0-200)		110 (6-240)	22 (0-43)		
279	Sausages, Spanish botifarra catalana		0 (0-1.8)		5.1 (4.0-22.0)			
280	Sausages, Spanish chorizo		17.5 (0-314.3)		282.3 (29.2-626.8)	15.9 (0-87.8)		

No	Name	Detail	Histamine	Phenyl-ethylamine	Tyramine	Tryptamine	Serotonine	Ethylamine
281	Sausages, Spanish Chouriça de Vinhais		1.6		75.9			
282	Sausages, Spanish fuet		15.2		156.9	10		
283	Sausages, Spanish fuet		2.2 (0-57.7)		190.7 (31.8-742.6)	8.7 (0-67.8)		
284	Sausages, Spanish Salpicão de Vinhais		0.2		13.4			
285	Sausages, Spanish salsichon		19.4		198.4	21.3		
286	Sausages, Spanish salsichon		7.3 (0-150.9)		280.5 (53.3-513.4)	8.5 (0-65.1)		
287	Sausages, Spanish sobrasada		9.0 (2.8-143.1)		332.1 (57.6-500.6)	11.5 (0-64.8)		
288	Sausages, Spanish thin fuet		1.8		121.8	6.5		
289	Sausages, Spanish, Chorizo, high pressure	Spain	0.9		19			
290	Sausages, Spanish, Chorizo, non-packed	Spain	16		215			
291	Sausages, Spanish, Chorizo, protective atmosphere packed	Spain	0.5		153			
292	Sausages, Spanish, cooked white, Butifarra, high pressure	Spain	0.4		0.5			
293	Sausages, Spanish, cooked white, Butifarra, vacuum packed	Spain	0.8		6			
294	Sausages, Turkish sucuk		12.5		167.6			
295	Smoked meat				471			
296	Smoked sausage		3	3	85			
298	Turkey, breast	Spain	0.04		5			
299	Turkey, breast, prepared with mushrooms	Spain	<DL		5			
300	NUTS & SEEDS							
301	Almond						1	

No	Name	Detail	Histamine	Phenyl-ethylamine	Tyramine	Tryptamine	Serotonine	Ethylamine
303	Beech nut						1	
305	Cashew nut						1	
307	Coconut						1	
309	Hazelnut		0		0		2	
312	Paranut						1	
313	Peanut		0		0			
316	Pecan nut						33	
325	Walnut						107	
328	VEGETABLES							
334	Bamboo sprouts		0	0	11	0		
335	Beet		4		13			
338	Belgian endive		0		0			
339	Broccoli		0		0		0	
341	Brussels sprouts		0		0			
343	Cabbage		1		1			
344	Cabbage, Chinese	5 days, 5°C	0.9		2.1			
347	Carrot		0		0			
349	Cauliflower		0		(400)		0	
351	Celeriac / celery root		0		0			
352	Celery		0		0			
359	Cucumber		0		(250)			
362	Eggplant		38		61	3	(2)	
365	Endive	5 days, 5°C	0		2.0			
366	Endive		0		2			
371	Kale or borecole		2		0			
372	Kohlrabi				(1400)			
373	Leek		0		12			
375	Lettuce / Iceberg lettuce		0		1			
377	Lettuce, Iceberg		0		1.8			
380	Mushroom, common		0		6			
382	Mushroom, Oyster		0		0			
386	Olives, black, green		0		0		0.2	
388	Onions		0		11			
397	Potatoes		1		8		58	
399	Radicchio	5 days, 5°C	0		1.8			
400	Radish		0		3			
403	Sauerkraut		38.0 (1.0-104)		75.0 (2.0-192)			
404	Sauerkraut		85	9	138			
405	Sauerkraut, -ecological		116		155			
406	Sauerkraut, -spices		46		143			
407	Sauerkraut, -wine		104		165			
409	Spinach		26		4		0	
410	Spinach leaves		61		<DL		<DL	

No	Name	Detail	Histamine	Phenyl-ethylamine	Tyramine	Tryptamine	Serotonine	Ethylamine
411	Spinach leaves, frozen		12					
413	Spinach, frozen		0		0			
415	Spinach, stored at 4°C for 3 weeks		<DL					
418	Sweet pepper / Bell pepper		0		8			
422	Tomato ketchup		4					
439	Tomatoes		4		0		4	4
440	Tomatoes		4					
441	Turnip tops / Turnip greens		2		0			
443	Verdolaga / Pigweed / little Hogweed / Pusley		2		0			
446	LEGUMES / BEANS & PRODUCTS							
449	Bean, Mung-, sprouts		0		0			
454	Beans, common		0		0			
455	Beans, Green / beans, French / beans, Runner		0		(230)			
461	Beans, White-, in tomato-sauce		0		0			
464	Miso, retail market		7.7 (0-102)		16 (0-49)	49 (0-762)		
465	Miso, supermarket		16 (0-221)		12 (0-28)	27 (0-434)		
466	Nattō, Japanese (fermented soybeans)		35 (0-457)		1.2 (0-45)	9.1 (301)		
467	Nattō, Taiwanese (fermented soybeans)		45 (0-137)		0	0		
468	Pea, Snow-		0		0			
469	Peas		0		0			
474	Sauce for Sashimi, Chao Shi Fa		633					
475	Soy sauce		2	0	882	100		
476	Soy sauce, Chinese		0-592		0-673			
477	Soy sauce, First Class soy sauce, Mong go		73					
478	Soy sauce, Superior light soy sauce, Hay Tian Brand		641					
479	Soy sauce, Tamari		2121					
480	Sufu, brown (fermened		2.7 (0-15.8)		1.1 (0-6.5)	0		

No	Name	Detail	Histamine	Phenyl-ethylamine	Tyramine	Tryptamine	Serotonine	Ethylamine
	soybean curd)							
481	Sufu, white (fermented soybean curd)		4.6 (0-20)		8 (0-40)	16 (0-81)		
482	Tempeh		185	0	150	0		
483	Tofu		1		0			
484	CEREALS / GRAINS & PRODUCTS							
490	Maize		1	4	1			
491	Maize, fresh		0.4		7.4			
505	Sourdough bread		0		0			
512	Wheat germ		2		0			
514	FRUIT & PRODUCTS							
515	Apple and juice				0			
525	Avocado		0		0		2	
527	Banana		0		0	1	22	
545	Dates		0		0		1	
548	Fig						0	
552	Grapefruit and juice		0	0	0		1	
555	Grapes and juice		1	1	0	0	0	
565	Kiwi fruit		0		0			
566	Kiwi fruit		2		<DL		9.2	
568	Kiwi fruit, stored at 4°C for 2 weeks		<DL					
569	Lemon juice		0	0	0			
574	Mandarin orange and juice		0	0	1			
578	Watermelon		0		(460)			
581	Orange and juice		1	0	0		0	
584	Papaya							
585	Passion fruit						(4)	
591	Pear				(0)			
597	Pineapple		0		0		22	
602	Plum, blue and red				6	5	10	
609	Raisins				0			
612	Raspberry and juice		0	2	93			
613	Raspberry marmalade		0		38			
615	Strawberry		0	0	0			
674	ALCOHOLIC DRINKS							
677	Beer		<1		<1			
678	Beer, alcohol-free		0	1	2	2		

No	Name	Detail	Histamine	Phenyl-ethylamine	Tyramine	Tryptamine	Serotonine	Ethylamine
679	Beer, Brazilian		0.2 (<0.2-1.5)		2.2 (0.3-36.8)	0.5 (<0.35-10.1)		
680	Beer, Kriek and Geuze		16		36			
681	Beer, Lager		0.72					
682	Beer, pilsener / pilsner		7	2	25	4		
686	Beer, wheat		0.57 (0.54-0.60)					
687	Brewer's yeast				478			
692	Ciders		1.1 (0.9-6.9)		1.3 (2.0-5.0)			
693	Ciders, natural from Spain and France		1.28		3.30			
700	Sherry		3 (0-9)		7 (0.5-17.0)			
710	Wine		1.5 (0-6)		1.3 (0-5)			
711	Wine, red		0.5-26.9		1.1-10.7			
713	Wine, red Barcelona				0.59			
714	Wine, red Cabernet Sauvignon		3.2 (0.8-5.5)					
715	Wine, red Rioja				4.20			
716	Wine, red, Spanish		4 (0-11)	0.1 (0-2)	1 (0-11)			
717	Wine, rose Castilla				0			
718	Wine, various		6	3	5			
719	Wine, white Cadiz				0			
720	Wine, white Pinot Grigio		0					
732	SUGAR & SWEETS							
735	Chocolate		1	10	8	10	18	
736	Chocolate, 70% cocoa		3.3		<DL		7.3	
737	Chocolate, dark		<DL		<DL		<DL	
738	Chocolate, milk		<DL		<DL		<DL	
742	Honey		1	1	0			
758	CONDIMENTS (SPICES, HERBS, SAUCES)							
769	Broth		6	0	0			
809	Mustard		0		0			
837	Vinegar		2	0	4			
838	Vinegar, balsamic		1.5					
840	Vinegar, red wine		0.1					
843	Yeast extract, Marmite		83	8	645			

No	Name	Detail	Histamine	Phenyl-ethylamine	Tyramine	Tryptamine	Serotonine	Ethylamine
873	FRAGRANCES, AROMAS, PERFUMES							
874	Aroma		8	0	10			

<DL: less than detection limit
():   less reliable analysis method

1 ppm = 1 mg/kg
mg/l ≈ mg/kg

The ALBA 1996 list gives Tryptophan concentrations but we have assumed it is tryptamine because tryptophan is an amino acid and not an amine. This needs to be checked!

Table 28 Biogenic amine concentrations in food

Concentrations in mg/kg.

No	Name	Detail	Putrescine	Cadaverine	Spermidine	Spermine	Agmatine	Reference BA
			mg/kg	mg/kg	mg/kg	mg/kg	mg/kg	.
65	DAIRY							.
66	Año, Spanish cheese							Izquierdo2003
67	Azeitão, Portuguese sheep cheese, raw milk		110-137	161-231				Pinho2001
68	Blue cheeses		18.0 (3.0-257.2)	11.3 (0-2101.4)	10.1 (0-71.6)	0 (0-18.9)	1.1 (0-28.5)	Novella-Rodriguez2003
70	Blue vein cheese, pasteurized milk	7 weeks ripening	<DL-117	3-491				Komprda2008
71	Blue-veined cheese		52.2 (10.1-60.4)	90.2 (12.2-190.7)	11.8 (6.2-17.2)	0.6 (0-1.1)		Marino2000
72	Brie cheese		5	2				ALBA1996
73	Brie cheese from farmhouse		619	1545				ALBA1996
74	Camembert cheese		300	480				ALBA1996
75	Camembert cheese from farmhouse		469	1530				ALBA1996
77	Castelmagno			310.4	0.42	449.6		Gosetti2007
78	Cheddar cheese		370	240				ALBA1996
79	Cheddar cheese	Egypt		10				Ibrahim2010
82	Cheddar cheese, ripened		650					Bardócz1993
83	Cheddar cheese, young		10-20					Bardócz1993
84	Cottage cheese							ALBA1996
86	Danish blue (Danablu) cheese		145	13				ALBA1996
87	Dutch cheese		19.0 (1.0-71.0)	73.0 (1.0-140.0)				ten Brink1990
88	Dutch-type cheese, hard, pasteurized milk	22 weeks ripening	6-61	1-2				Komprda2007
89	Dutch-type cheese, semihard, pasteurized milk	25 weeks ripening	1-132					Komprda2008
90	Edam cheese, young		18	17				ALBA1996
91	Egyptian blue cheese							Rabie2011
92	Emmentaler cheese		211	79				ALBA1996

No	Name	Detail	Putrescine	Cadaverine	Spermidine	Spermine	Agmatine	Reference BA
93	Feta cheese		0	7				ALBA1996
94	Feta cheese, Greek goat/sheep, brined, thermized milk	17 weeks ripening	193	83				Valsamaki2000
95	Goat cheese		61	134				ALBA1996
96	Goat cheese	13 weeks ripening	34	4				Novella2002
97	Goat cheese, raw milk	13 weeks ripening	86-175	196-314				Novella2004
98	Goat cheeses		4.1 (0-191.8)	0.7 (0-88.7)	0.9 (0-14.5)	0 (0-3.6)	0 (0-3.2)	Novella-Rodriguez2003
99	Gorgonzola cheese		680	2805				ALBA1996
100	Gouda cheese		265	193				ALBA1996
101	Gouda cheese	Egypt		5				Ibrahim2010
102	Gouda cheese	12 weeks ripening	4-42					Leuschner1998
103	Grana Padano cheese	Italy						Coïsson2008
104	Grana type cheese	Italy						Coïsson2008
105	Gruyère cheese		10	29				ALBA1996
106	Hard-ripened cheese from pasteurized milk		5.0 (0-611.7)	8.0 (0-710.1)	5.7 (0-43.0)	1.6 (0-18.7)	0 (0-22.0)	Novella-Rodriguez2003
107	Hard-ripened cheese from raw milk		8.1 (0-62.5)	29.5 (0.9-368.5)	0.1 (0-39.6)	0 (0-21.5)	0 (0-27.2)	Novella-Rodriguez2003
108	Maasdam cheese		3542	1142				ALBA1996
109	Manchego, Spanish cheese							Izquierdo2003
110	Mascarpone		618	1658				ALBA1996
113	Mozzarella		0	0				ALBA1996
114	Parmesan cheese		43	98				ALBA1996
115	Parmesan cheese							Izquierdo2003
116	Parmigiano Reggiano cheese							Coïsson2008
117	Pecorino di Farindola cheese	90 days ripening, Italy, 10 farms	10-394	27-276	25-144			Schirone2011
118	Processed cheese		4-60	12-120				El-Sayed1996
119	Processed cheese		1-2	1				Komprda2005
120	Raclette cheese							Schmutz2006
121	Ras, Egyptian cheese	Egypt		8				Ibrahim2010
122	Raschera			118.9	10.6	352.7		Gosetti2007
123	Roquefort cheese		107	617				ALBA1996

No	Name	Detail	Putrescine	Cadaverine	Spermidine	Spermine	Agmatine	Reference BA
124	Semihard Italian cheese, unpasteurized milk	21 weeks ripening	129-1105	5-30				Innocente2002
125	Semisoft cheese, pasteurized milk	20 weeks ripening	1-13	6-109				Schneller1997
126	Semisoft cheese, raw milk	20 weeks ripening	76-308	280-2369				Schneller1997
127	Sheep cheese		375	1274				ALBA1996
128	Sheep cheese, Portuguese, traditional, raw milk	9 weeks ripening	218	207				Pinho2004
129	Spanish retail cheeses, ripened		<DL-612	4-215				Novella2000
130	Spanish retail cheeses, unripened		<DL-1	<1				Novella2000
131	Spanish traditional cheeses							Roig2002
132	Spreadable cheese, Dutch		0	44				ALBA1996
133	Spreadable cheese, non-Dutch		21	51				ALBA1996
134	Swiss cheese		600	680				ALBA1996
135	Swiss-type cheese	24 weeks ripening	17-360	17-360				Petridis1999
136	Tilsiter cheese		313	147				ALBA1996
137	Toma piemontese			1.3	6.6	193.9		Gosetti2007
138	Unripened cheese		0 (0-3.1)	0 (0-1.5)	0.3 (0-0.8)	0- (0-1.1)	0	Novella-Rodriguez2003
140	Yogurt		<1	<1				ten Brink1990
141	SEAFOOD & PRODUCTS							
142	Anchovy paste		37	184				ALBA1996
143	Anchovy sauce							Lauryssen2005
144	Anchovy, canned		60	225				ALBA1996
145	Anchovy, canned	Taiwan	14 (0-34)	13 (0-28)	4 (0-8)	21 (0-47)	0	Tsai2005
146	Anchovy, fresh, summer	Taiwan						Yeh2004
147	Anchovy, fresh, winter	Taiwan						Yeh2004
148	Anchovy, salt ripened		10.7 (6.5-17.2)	20.7 (7.1-47.8)			27.7 (12.7-57.5)	Pons2005
149	Bloater (herring)		61	0				ALBA1996
150	Bonito, canned	Taiwan	3 (0-15)	8 (0-18)	4 (0-6)	24 (0-53)	0	Tsai2005
151	Cod		14	34				ALBA1996
152	Crab		0	0				ALBA1996

No	Name	Detail	Putrescine	Cadaverine	Spermidine	Spermine	Agmatine	Reference BA
154	Eel, fresh and fumed		0	0				ALBA1996
156	Fish meal, dried		546	992				denBrinker1995
157	Fish paste		12 (5.0-17)	58 (22-107)				Tsai2006
158	Fish sauce		24 (2.0-243)	89 (0-243)				Tsai2006
159	Fish sauce, from Far East		0-1257	0-1429				Stute2002
160	Fish, canned		7	6				denBrinker1995
161	Haddock liver		73	51				ALBA1996
162	Haddock, fresh and frozen		0	0				ALBA1996
163	Haddock, fumed		24	77				ALBA1996
164	Hake, fresh		3	0.5	3		0.3	Ruiz2001
165	Herring, in tomato sauce		12	50				ALBA1996
166	Herring, pickled							ALBA1996
167	Herring, salted		35	64				ALBA1996
168	Herring, vinegar		10	33				ALBA1996
169	Mackerel, canned		227	540				ALBA1996
170	Mackerel, canned	Taiwan	6 (0-21)	6 (0-26)	2 (0-5)	46 (0-251)	0	Tsai2005
171	Mackerel, fresh		55	49				ALBA1996
172	Mackerel, fresh, summer	Taiwan						Yeh2004
173	Mackerel, fresh, winter	Taiwan						Yeh2004
174	Mackerel, fumed		16	221				ALBA1996
175	Mackerel, salted, retail market	Northern Taiwan	1.9 (0-5.9)	2.1 (0-26.0)	3.9 (0-42.0)	21.4 (0-66.5)	1.2 (0-8.0)	Tsai2005
176	Mackerel, salted, retail market	Southern Taiwan	2.3 (0-2.4)	5.7 (0-18.3)	5.3 (0-52.1)	26.9 (0-54.5)	1.5 (0-9.2)	Tsai2005
177	Mackerel, salted, supermarket	Northern Taiwan	1.4 (0-9.8)	5.0 (0-21.0)	0	28.9 (0-84.1)	1.4 (0-3.5)	Tsai2005
178	Mackerel, salted, supermarket	Southern Taiwan	0	1.6 (0-1.2)?	1.3 (0-14.1)	21.2 (0-46.0)	1.7 (0-2.6)	Tsai2005
179	Marlin, fresh, summer	Taiwan						Yeh2004
180	Marlin, fresh, winter	Taiwan						Yeh2004
181	Milk fish, canned	Taiwan	2 (0-5)	1 (0-4)	1 (0-2)	0	0	Tsai2005
182	Mussels: fresh, vinegar and canned		1	2				ALBA1996
184	Pacific saury, canned	Taiwan	4 (0-10)	10 (0-22)	0	15 (0-27)	0	Tsai2005
185	Plaice, fresh and baked		2	1				ALBA1996
186	Pollock		21	0				ALBA1996
188	Salmon, canned		173	108				ALBA1996

No	Name	Detail	Putrescine	Cadaverine	Spermidine	Spermine	Agmatine	Reference BA
189	Salmon, fresh		11	19				ALBA1996
191	Salmon, smoked		53	550				ALBA1996
192	Sardines, canned		43	60				ALBA1996
195	Shrimp paste		40 (5-118)	80 (0-162)				Tsai2006
196	Shrimps		11	5				ALBA1996
197	Sprat, canned		0	72				ALBA1996
198	Tarasi (shrimp paste)		6395	7455				ALBA1996
199	Trout rainbow, fresh		0.42	0.17				Rezaei2007
200	Trout, smoked		0	300				ALBA1996
201	Tub Gurnard / Tom Grimard		4	38				ALBA1996
202	Tuna, canned		2	10				ALBA1996
203	Tuna, canned	Taiwan	8 (0-35)	4 (0-28)	3 (0-4)	41 (0-202)	1 (0-3)	Tsai2005
204	Tuna, fresh		0	0				ALBA1996
205	Tuna, fresh, red muscle		3.0	1.0	42.5		0.2	Ruiz2004
206	Tuna, fresh, white muscle		4.5	2.4	21.8		3.1	Ruiz2004
208	Whiting		28	41				ALBA1996
209	**MEAT & EGG**							
210	Alheira, Portugese smoked fermented sausage		0-6.2	0-39.7				Ferreira2006
212	Bovine meat		2.1	18.5	2.2	17.2		Vinci2002
213	Chicken liver							ALBA1996
214	Chicken meat		27	9				ALBA1996
216	Cow liver							ALBA1996
217	Cow meat		8	8				ALBA1996
218	Cow meat, chopped		9	105				ALBA1996
219	Deli sandwich (cooked product of meat and salmon)	Spain	0.2	0.2				Ruiz2004
223	Ham meat, cooked		565	245				ALBA1996
224	Ham, cooked		0 (0-12.4)	0.4 (0-9.5)	2.1 (1.4-3.5)	21.4 (6.4-35.7)		Hernandez-Jover1997
225	Ham, cooked with fibre (Bioyork)	Spain	2	0.4				Ruiz2004
226	Ham, cooked, sliced, high pressure	Spain	1	8				Ruiz2004
227	Ham, cooked, sliced, protective atmophere packed	Spain	4	44				Ruiz2004
228	Ham, cooked, sliced, vacuum packed	Spain	8	5				Ruiz2004

No	Name	Detail	Putrescine	Cadaverine	Spermidine	Spermine	Agmatine	Reference BA
229	Ham, cured, sliced, protective atmosphere packed	Spain	0.2	6				Ruiz2004
230	Ham, cured, sliced, vacuum packed	Spain	1	6				Ruiz2004
231	Ham, dry-cured, Italian	15 months old	0.13 (0-2.0)	0.30 (0-2.0)	7.8 (2.0-19)	42.1 (21-67)		Virgili2007
232	Ham, dry-cured, Italian	23 months old	72.3 (19.0-218)	5.5 (1.0-15)	4.4 (0-11)			Virgili2007
233	Ham, dry-cured, Spanish		2.3 (0-17.4)	2.1 (0-305.5)	5.6 (4.4-7.3)	35.7 (24.9-62.1)		Hernandez-Jover1997
234	Ham, raw		598	97				ALBA1996
235	Hare liver		352	858				ALBA1996
236	Hare meat		70	219				ALBA1996
239	Liver sausage		0	0				ALBA1996
241	Loin, pickled, non-packed	Spain	Nd	6				Ruiz2004
242	Loin, pickled, protective atmosphere packed	Spain	0.2	7				Ruiz2004
243	Loin, steak, non-packed	Spain	0.3	0.5				Ruiz2004
244	Loin, steak, protective atmosphere packed	Spain	0.1	0.1				Ruiz2004
245	Meat extract, dry		17	21				ALBA1996
246	Mortadella, Spanish		1.3 (0-5.7)	1.7 (4.3-28.8)?	4.0 (1.0-8.9)	17.2 (7.6-32.2)		Hernandez-Jover1997
247	Poličane		54 (54-54)	6 (6-6)	2.5 (2-3)	2 (2-2)		Komprda2001
248	Pork meat		9	13				ALBA1996
249	Pork meat chopped		69	96				ALBA1996
253	Sausage, dry (various)		145	137				ALBA1996
254	Sausage, Dutch, dry, Rotterdammer		160	33				ALBA1996
255	Sausage, ripened fermented	France	0-362	0-390				Latorre2008
256	Sausage, ripened fermented	Greece	0-126	0-243				Latorre2008
257	Sausage, ripened fermented	Italy	4-324	0-449				Latorre2008
258	Sausage, ripened fermented	Portugal	4-352	3-485				Latorre2008
259	Sausage, ripened fermented	Slovakia	0-62	0-3				Latorre2008
260	Sausage,	Spain	1-449	0-611				Latorre2008

No	Name	Detail	Putrescine	Cadaverine	Spermidine	Spermine	Agmatine	Reference BA
	ripened fermented							
261	Sausages, Belgian		15.1 (3.1-40)	2.5 (0-5.6)				Vandekerckhove1977
262	Sausages, Belgian North		33	0	3	12		Ansorena2002
263	Sausages, Belgian South		125	5	4	15		Ansorena2002
264	Sausages, Danish		130 (0-450)	180 (0-790)	7 (3-9)	37 (23-47)		Eerola1998
265	Sausages, Egyptian		39 (12-100)	19 (5.6-39)	2.3 (5.3-12)	1.8 (1.5-5.3)		Shalaby1993
266	Sausages, fermented		52 (1-190)	63 (1-150)				tenBrink1990
267	Sausages, Finnish		79 (0-230)	50 (0-270)	4 (2-7)	31 (19-46)		Eerola1998
268	Sausages, French saucisson, industrial		279 (195-410)	103 (31-192)	5.1 (4-6.4)	91 (59-119)		Montel 1999
269	Sausages, French saucisson, traditional		223 (61-317)	71.3 (39-110)	4.3 (2-6)	83.7 (82-86)		Montel 1999
270	Sausages, German Mettwurst		77 (2-580)	6 (0-16)	6 (3-11)	29 (22-38)		Eerola1998
271	Sausages, Italian		1	1	6	18		Ansorena2002
272	Sausages, Italian salsiccia		19.7 (0-77.7)	6.7 (0-39)	18.8 (0-57.2)	2.8 (0-28.1)		Parente2001
273	Sausages, Italian, Salami, Soppressata	Italy	98.8 (0-416.1)	60.8 (0-271.4)	40 (0-91.3)	35.5 (0-97.9)		Parente2001
274	Sausages, Italian, Salamini italiani alla cacciatora PDO	Italy						Coïsson2004
275	Sausages, Norwegian		1	1	4	24		Ansorena2002
276	Sausages, Portugese Painho de Portalegre, 3% NaCl		1047.5	1732.1	8.5	12.0		Roseiro2006
277	Sausages, Portugese Painho de Portalegre, 6% NaCl		601.4	295.6	17.5	29.6		Roseiro2006
278	Sausages, Russian		93 (3-310)	10 (3-18)	5 (2-8)	33 (23-40)		Eerola1998
279	Sausages, Spanish botifarra catalana		0.7 (0-3.7)	9.6 (0-40.0)	2.9 (1.2-5.3)	17.9 (12.5-25.8)		Hernandez-Jover1997)
280	Sausages, Spanish chorizo		60.4 (2.6-415.6)	20.1 (0-658.1)				Hernandez-Jover1997)
281	Sausages, Spanish		11.3	1.7				Ferreira2007

No	Name	Detail	Putrescine	Cadaverine	Spermidine	Spermine	Agmatine	Reference BA
	Chouriça de Vinhais							
282	Sausages, Spanish fuet		64.7	367.2	10.3	30.6		Bover-Cid1999
283	Sausages, Spanish fuet		71.6 (2.2-222.1)	18.9 (5.4-51.3)				Hernandez-Jover1997)
284	Sausages, Spanish Salpicão de Vinhais		0.4	0.1				Ferreira2007
285	Sausages, Spanish salsichon		138.5	26.4	5.6	35.2		Bover-Cid1999
286	Sausages, Spanish salsichon		102.7 (5.5-400)	11.7 (0-342.3)				Hernandez-Jover1997)
287	Sausages, Spanish sobrasada		65.2 (1.8-500.7)	12.6 (3.0-41.6)				Hernandez-Jover1997)
288	Sausages, Spanish thin fuet		105.2	56.3	9.2	32.8		Bover-Cid1999
289	Sausages, Spanish, Chorizo, high pressure	Spain	0.8	9				Ruiz2004
290	Sausages, Spanish, Chorizo, non-packed	Spain	185	229				Ruiz2004
291	Sausages, Spanish, Chorizo, protective atmosphere packed	Spain	89	71				Ruiz2004
292	Sausages, Spanish, cooked white, Butifarra, high pressure	Spain	0.2	0.07				Ruiz2004
293	Sausages, Spanish, cooked white, Butifarra, vacuum packed	Spain	10	40				Ruiz2004
294	Sausages, Turkish sucuk		82.7	33.2	14.6	54.6		Genccelep2007
295	Smoked meat							ALBA1996
296	Smoked sausage		136	37				ALBA1996
298	Turkey, breast	Spain	0.4	3				Ruiz2004
299	Turkey, breast, prepared with mushrooms	Spain	0.8	1				Ruiz2004
300	NUTS & SEEDS							
301	Almond							ALBA1996
303	Beech nut							ALBA1996
305	Cashew nut							ALBA1996
307	Coconut							ALBA1996

No	Name	Detail	Putrescine	Cadaverine	Spermidine	Spermine	Agmatine	Reference BA
309	Hazelnut		0	0				ALBA1996
312	Paranut							ALBA1996
313	Peanut		0	0				ALBA1996
316	Pecan nut							ALBA1996
325	Walnut							ALBA1996
328	VEGETABLES							
334	Bamboo sprouts		2	0				ALBA1996
335	Beet		9	0				ALBA1996
338	Belgian endive		8	0				ALBA1996
339	Broccoli		32	0				ALBA1996
341	Brussels sprouts		0	0				ALBA1996
343	Cabbage		14	0				ALBA1996
344	Cabbage, Chinese	5 days, 5°C	11.3		11.7	0.27		Simon-Sarkadi1994
347	Carrot		8	0				ALBA1996
349	Cauliflower		1.0	0				ALBA1996
351	Celeriac / celery root		5	0				ALBA1996
352	Celery		6	0				ALBA1996
359	Cucumber		16	0				ALBA1996
362	Eggplant		0	0				ALBA1996
365	Endive	5 days, 5°C	9.9		7.4	0.16		Simon-Sarkadi1994
366	Endive		5	7				ALBA1996
371	Kale or borecole		15	0				ALBA1996
372	Kohlrabi							ALBA1996
373	Leek		39	0				ALBA1996
375	Lettuce / Iceberg lettuce		10	0				ALBA1996
377	Lettuce, Iceberg		15.7		6.1	0.16		Simon-Sarkadi1994
380	Mushroom, common		9	0				ALBA1996
382	Mushroom, Oyster		1	0				ALBA1996
386	Olives, black, green		0	0				ALBA1996
388	Onions		7	0				ALBA1996
397	Potatoes		4	0				ALBA1996
399	Radicchio	5 days, 5°C	14.4		10.1	0.27		Simon-Sarkadi1994
400	Radish		12	0				ALBA1996
403	Sauerkraut		154.0 (6.0-550)	73.0 (1.0-311)				ten Brink1990
404	Sauerkraut		396	91				ALBA1996
405	Sauerkraut, -ecological		343	89				ALBA1996
406	Sauerkraut, -spices		352	95				ALBA1996
407	Sauerkraut, -wine		365	94				ALBA1996
409	Spinach		8	0				ALBA1996
410	Spinach leaves		8	<DL				Dionex2007
411	Spinach leaves, frozen							Schmutz2006
413	Spinach, frozen		8	0				ALBA1996

No	Name	Detail	Putrescine	Cadaverine	Spermidine	Spermine	Agmatine	Reference BA
415	Spinach, stored at 4°C for 3 weeks		13	5				Dionex2007
418	Sweet pepper / Bell pepper		44	0				ALBA1996
422	Tomato ketchup							Schmutz2006
439	Tomatoes		26	0				ALBA1996
440	Tomatoes							Schmutz2006
441	Turnip tops / Turnip greens		2	0				ALBA1996
443	Verdolaga / Pigweed / little Hogweed / Pusley		12	5				ALBA1996
446	**LEGUMES / BEANS & PRODUCTS**							.
449	Bean, Mung-, sprouts		0	0				ALBA1996
454	Beans, common		0	0				ALBA1996
455	Beans, Green / beans, French / beans, Runner		12	0				ALBA1996
461	Beans, White-, in tomato-sauce		0	0				ALBA1996
464	Miso, retail market		1.1 (0-9)	9 (0-30)	0	7.2 (0-93)	5.8 (0-75)	Kung2007
465	Miso, supermarket		1.2 (0-12)	32 (0-201)	0	8 (0-216)	2.4 (0-66)	Kung2007
466	Nattō, Japanese (fermented soybeans)		17 (0-27)	22 (2-42)	45 (0-124)	8.6 (0-71)	0	Tsai2007
467	Nattō, Taiwanese (fermented soybeans)		1.6 (0-6)	0.5 (0-3)	25 (0-50)	0	0	Tsai2007
468	Pea, Snow-		0	0				ALBA1996
469	Peas		0	0				ALBA1996
474	Sauce for Sashimi, Chao Shi Fa							Lauryssen2005
475	Soy sauce		(80)	(200)				ALBA1996
476	Soy sauce, Chinese			0-550				Lu2009
477	Soy sauce, First Class soy sauce, Mong go							Lauryssen2005
478	Soy sauce, Superior light soy sauce, Hay Tian Brand							Lauryssen2005
479	Soy sauce, Tamari							ALBA1996
480	Sufu, brown (fermened soybean curd)		0.24 (0-1.0)	5.0 (0-37.1)	0	0		Kung2007
481	Sufu, white (fermented		15 (0-45)	7 (0-41)	0	16 (0-82)		Kung2007

No	Name	Detail	Putrescine	Cadaverine	Spermidine	Spermine	Agmatine	Reference BA
	soybean curd)							
482	Tempeh		500	617				ALBA1996
483	Tofu		4	1				ALBA1996
484	CEREALS / GRAINS & PRODUCTS							
490	Maize		78	0				ALBA1996
491	Maize, fresh		11.0	4.2				Nishino2007
505	Sourdough bread		0	0				ALBA1996
512	Wheat germ		140	2				ALBA1996
514	FRUIT & PRODUCTS							
515	Apple and juice							ALBA1996
525	Avocado		0	0				ALBA1996
527	Banana		60	0				ALBA1996
545	Dates		0	0				ALBA1996
548	Fig							ALBA1996
552	Grapefruit and juice		40	0				ALBA1996
555	Grapes and juice		3	0				ALBA1996
565	Kiwi fruit		0	0				ALBA1996
566	Kiwi fruit		3	<DL				Dionex2007
568	Kiwi fruit, stored at 4°C for 2 weeks		<DL	<DL				Dionex2007
569	Lemon juice		3	0				ALBA1996
574	Mandarin orange and juice		109	0				ALBA1996
578	Watermelon		0	0				ALBA1996
581	Orange and juice		53	0				ALBA1996
584	Papaya							ALBA1996
585	Passion fruit							ALBA1996
591	Pear							ALBA1996
597	Pineapple							ALBA1996
602	Plum, blue and red							ALBA1996
609	Raisins							ALBA1996
612	Raspberry and juice		13	0				ALBA1996
613	Raspberry marmalade		0	0				ALBA1996
615	Strawberry		4	0				ALBA1996
674	ALCOHOLIC DRINKS							
677	Beer		4 (0.5-8)	9.5 (0-60)				ten Brink1990
678	Beer, alcohol-free		3	0				ALBA1996
679	Beer, Brazilian		3.9 (0.9-9.8)	0.5 (<0.2-2.6)	0.7 (<0.2-6.0)		10.9 (2.1-46.8)	Gloria1999
680	Beer, Kriek and Geuze		17	19				ALBA1996

No	Name	Detail	Putrescine	Cadaverine	Spermidine	Spermine	Agmatine	Reference BA
681	Beer, Lager		3.0	0	0.14	0.33	14.9	De Borba 2007
682	Beer, pilsener / pilsner		8	34				ALBA1996
686	Beer, wheat		6.5 (6.4-6.6)	0.48 (0.28-0.67)	0.82 (0.45-1.20)	0.6 (0.47-0.73)	8.4 (7.7-9.1)	De Borba 2007
687	Brewer's yeast							ALBA1996
692	Ciders		3.6 (3.3-12.3)					Garai2006
693	Ciders, natural from Spain and France		3.49	2.74				Ladero2011
700	Sherry		9 (3-25)	<1				ten Brink1990
710	Wine		4 (1-12)	<1				ten Brink1990
711	Wine, red		2.9-122					Konakovsky2011
713	Wine, red Barcelona							Gil-Agusti2007
714	Wine, red Cabernet Sauvignon		13.3 (7.1-19.4)	0.66 (0.53-0.79)	1.7 (1.4-1.9)	0.2 (0.21-0.19)?	0.3 (0.23-0.37)	De Borba 2007
715	Wine, red Rioja							Gil-Agusti2007
716	Wine, red, Spanish		7 (0-27)	0.2 (0-3)				Marcobal2005
717	Wine, rose Castilla							Gil-Agusti2007
718	Wine, various		36	1				ALBA1996
719	Wine, white Cadiz							Gil-Agusti2007
720	Wine, white Pinot Grigio		1.7	0	0	0	0	De Borba2007
732	SUGAR & SWEETS							
735	Chocolate		2	2				ALBA1996
736	Chocolate, 70% cocoa		6.9	<DL				Dionex2007
737	Chocolate, dark		<DL	<DL				Dionex2007
738	Chocolate, milk		<DL	<DL				Dionex2007
742	Honey		1	1				ALBA1996
758	CONDIMENTS (SPICES, HERBS, SAUCES)							
769	Broth		17	4				ALBA1996
809	Mustard		0	0				ALBA1996
837	Vinegar		2	0				ALBA1996
838	Vinegar, balsamic							Schmutz2006
840	Vinegar, red wine							Schmutz2006
843	Yeast extract, Marmite		70	6				ALBA1996
873	FRAGRANCES, AROMAS, PERFUMES							
874	Aroma		17	4				ALBA1996

Table 29 Mast cell degranulators, salicylates and lectin activity in food

Concentrations in mg/kg.

No	Name	Mast cell degranulators	Salicylates	Reference Salicylates	Lectin activity
			mg/kg		
65	DAIRY				
69	Blue Vein cheese, fresh		0.5	Swain 1985	
76	Camembert cheese, fresh		0.1	Swain 1985	
80	Cheddar cheese (Tasty), fresh		0.0	Swain 1985	
81	Cheddar cheese, fresh		0.0	Swain 1985	
85	Cottage cheese, fresh		0.0	Swain 1985	
111	Milk, fresh full cream, liquid		0.0	Swain 1985	
112	Mozarella cheese, fresh		0.2	Swain 1985	
139	Yoghurt, full cream, fresh		0.0	Swain 1985	
141	SEAFOOD & PRODUCTS				
153	Crustaceans	Schmutz2006			
183	Oyster, fresh		0.0	Swain 1985	
187	Prawn, fresh		0.4	Swain 1985	
190	Salmon, Lunchtime Pink, canned		0.0	Swain 1985	
193	Scallop, fresh		0.2	Swain 1985	
194	Shellfish	Schmutz2006			
207	Tuna, Seakist, canned		0.0	Swain 1985	
209	MEAT & EGG				
211	Beef, fresh		0.0	Swain 1985	
215	Chicken, fresh		0.0	Swain 1985	
220	Egg white	Vlieg2005, Schmutz2006, Maintz2007			
221	Egg, white, fresh		0.0	Swain 1985	
222	Egg, yolk, fresh		0.0	Swain 1985	
237	Kidney, fresh		0.0	Swain 1985	
238	Lamb, fresh		0.0	Swain 1985	
240	Liver, fresh		0.5	Swain 1985	
248	Pork meat	Vlieg2005, Maintz2007			
250	Pork, fresh		0.0	Swain 1985	
297	Tripe, fresh		0.0	Swain 1985	
300	NUTS & SEEDS	Vlieg2005, Schmutz2006 (especially rancid nuts), Maintz2007			
302	Almonds, fresh		30.0	Swain 1985	
304	Brazil nuts, fresh		4.6	Swain 1985	
306	Cashew nuts, fresh		0.7	Swain 1985	
308	Coconut, dessicated, dry		2.6	Swain 1985	Sharon 2007
310	Hazelnuts, fresh		1.4	Swain 1985	Sharon 2007
311	Macadamia nuts, fresh		5.2	Swain 1985	
314	Peanuts, Sanitarium butter, paste	Vlieg2005, Maintz2007	2.3	Swain 1985	
315	Peanuts, unshelled,	Vlieg2005,	11.2	Swain 1985	

No	Name	Mast cell degranulators	Salicylates	Reference Salicylates	Lectin activity
	fresh	Maintz2007			
317	Pecan nuts, fresh		1.2	Swain 1985	
318	Pine nuts, fresh		5.1	Swain 1985	
319	Pistachio nuts, fresh		5.5	Swain 1985	
320	Poppyseed, dry		0.0	Swain 1985	
321	Sesame seed, dry		2.3	Swain 1985	Sharon 2007
323	Sunflower seed, dry	Schmutz2006	1.2	Swain 1985	Sharon 2007
326	Walnuts, fresh		3.0	Swain 1985	
327	Water chestnut, Socomin, canned		29.2	Swain 1985	
328	VEGETABLES	.		.	.
329	Alfalfa				Sharon 2007
331	Asparagus, fresh		1.4	Swain 1985	Sharon 2007
332	Asparagus, Triangle Spears, canned		3.2	Swain 1985	Sharon 2007
333	Bamboo shoots, Sunshine, canned		0.0	Swain 1985	
336	Beetroot, fresh		1.8	Swain 1985	Sharon 2007
337	Beetroot, Golden Circle, canned		3.2	Swain 1985	Sharon 2007
340	Broccoli, fresh		6.5	Swain 1985	
342	Brussels sprouts, fresh		0.7	Swain 1985	
345	Cabbage, green, fresh		0.0	Swain 1985	
346	Cabbage, red, fresh		0.8	Swain 1985	
348	Carrot, fresh		2.3	Swain 1985	
350	Cauliflower, fresh		1.6	Swain 1985	
353	Celery, fresh		0.0	Swain 1985	Sharon 2007
355	Chicory, fresh		10.2	Swain 1985	
356	Chives, fresh		0.3	Swain 1985	
357	Choko, (Chayote), fresh		0.1	Swain 1985	
360	Cucumber, (no peel), fresh		7.8	Swain 1985	Sharon 2007
361	Cucumber, Aristocrate gherkin, canned		61.4	Swain 1985	Sharon 2007
363	Eggplant, (no peel), fresh		3.0	Swain 1985	
364	Eggplant, (with peel), fresh		8.8	Swain 1985	
367	Endive, fresh		19.0	Swain 1985	
370	Horseradish, Eskal, canned		1.8	Swain 1985	
374	Leek, , fresh		0.8	Swain 1985	
376	Lettuce, fresh		0.0	Swain 1985	
378	Marrow, (Cucurbita pepo), fresh		1.7	Swain 1985	
379	Mushroom, Champignon, canned		12.6	Swain 1985	
381	Mushroom, fresh		2.4	Swain 1985	Sharon 2007
383	Okra, Zanae, canned		5.9	Swain 1985	
384	Olive, black Kraft, canned		3.4	Swain 1985	
385	Olive, green Kraft, canned		12.9	Swain 1985	

No	Name	Mast cell degranulators	Salicylates	Reference Salicylates	Lectin activity
387	Onion, fresh		1.6	Swain 1985	
389	Parsnip, fresh		4.5	Swain 1985	
390	Peppers, green chili, fresh		6.4	Swain 1985	
391	Peppers, red chili, fresh		12.0	Swain 1985	
392	Peppers, sweet, green (Capsicum), fresh		12.0	Swain 1985	
393	Peppers, yello-green chili, fresh		6.2	Swain 1985	
394	Pimientos, Arson sweet red, canned		1.5	Swain 1985	
395	Potato, white (no peel), fresh		0.0	Swain 1985	Sharon 2007
396	Potato, white (with peel), fresh		1.2	Swain 1985	Sharon 2007
398	Pumpkin, fresh		1.2	Swain 1985	
401	Radish, red, small, fresh		12.4	Swain 1985	
408	Shallots, fresh		0.3	Swain 1985	
412	Spinach, fresh	Vlieg2005, Maintz2007	5.8	Swain 1985	
414	Spinach, frozen	Vlieg2005, Maintz2007	1.6	Swain 1985	
416	Squash, baby, fresh		6.3	Swain 1985	
417	Swede, fresh		0.0	Swain 1985	
420	Sweet potato, white, fresh		5.0	Swain 1985	Sharon 2007
421	Sweet potato, yellow, fresh		4.8	Swain 1985	Sharon 2007
423	Tomato, Campbell, paste	Vlieg2005, Schmutz2006, Maintz2007	5.7	Swain 1985	Sharon 2007
424	Tomato, Fountain, sauce	Vlieg2005, Schmutz2006, Maintz2007	9.4	Swain 1985	Sharon 2007
425	Tomato, fresh	Vlieg2005, Schmutz2006, Maintz2007	1.3	Swain 1985	Sharon 2007
426	Tomato, Goulbum Valley, juice	Vlieg2005, Schmutz2006, Maintz2007	1.0	Swain 1985	Sharon 2007
427	Tomato, Heinz, juice	Vlieg2005, Schmutz2006, Maintz2007	1.2	Swain 1985	Sharon 2007
428	Tomato, Heinz, sauce	Vlieg2005, Schmutz2006, Maintz2007	24.8	Swain 1985	Sharon 2007
429	Tomato, Heinz, soup	Vlieg2005, Schmutz2006, Maintz2007	5.4	Swain 1985	Sharon 2007
430	Tomato, I.X.L., sauce	Vlieg2005, Schmutz2006, Maintz2007	10.6	Swain 1985	Sharon 2007
431	Tomato, Kiaora, soup	Vlieg2005, Schmutz2006, Maintz2007	5.4	Swain 1985	Sharon 2007
432	Tomato, Leggo, paste	Vlieg2005, Schmutz2006, Maintz2007	14.4	Swain 1985	Sharon 2007
433	Tomato, Letona, canned	Vlieg2005, Schmutz2006, Maintz2007	5.3	Swain 1985	Sharon 2007

No	Name	Mast cell degranulators	Salicylates	Reference Salicylates	Lectin activity
434	Tomato, Letona, juice	Vlieg2005, Schmutz2006, Maintz2007	1.8	Swain 1985	Sharon 2007
435	Tomato, P.M.U., sauce	Vlieg2005, Schmutz2006, Maintz2007	9.8	Swain 1985	Sharon 2007
436	Tomato, P.M.U., soup	Vlieg2005, Schmutz2006, Maintz2007	3.2	Swain 1985	Sharon 2007
437	Tomato, Rosella, sauce	Vlieg2005, Schmutz2006, Maintz2007	21.5	Swain 1985	Sharon 2007
438	Tomato, Tom Piper, paste	Vlieg2005, Schmutz2006, Maintz2007	4.3	Swain 1985	Sharon 2007
442	Turnip, fresh		1.6	Swain 1985	
444	Watercress, fresh		8.4	Swain 1985	
445	Zucchini, fresh		10.4	Swain 1985	
446	LEGUMES / BEANS & PRODUCTS		.		Sharon 2007
447	Alfalfa, fresh		7.0	Swain 1985	Sharon 2007
448	Bean sprouts, fresh		0.6	Swain 1985	Sharon 2007
450	Beans, blackeye, dried		0.0	Swain 1985	Sharon 2007
451	Beans, Borlotti, dried		0.8	Swain 1985	Sharon 2007
452	Beans, broad, "vicia faba", fresh		7.3	Swain 1985	Sharon 2007
453	Beans, brown, dried		0.0	Swain 1985	Sharon 2007
456	Beans, green French, fresh		1.1	Swain 1985	Sharon 2007
457	Beans, lima, dried		0.0	Swain 1985	Sharon 2007
458	Beans, mung, dried		0.0	Swain 1985	Sharon 2007
459	Beans, soya grits, dried		0.0	Swain 1985	Sharon 2007
460	Beans, soya, dried		0.0	Swain 1985	Sharon 2007
462	Lentil, brown, dried		0.0	Swain 1985	Sharon 2007
463	Lentil, red, dried		0.0	Swain 1985	Sharon 2007
470	Peas, chick-pea, dried		0.0	Swain 1985	Sharon 2007
471	Peas, green split pea, dried		0.0	Swain 1985	Sharon 2007
472	Peas, green, fresh		0.4	Swain 1985	Sharon 2007
473	Peas, yellow split pea, dried		0.2	Swain 1985	Sharon 2007
484	CEREALS / GRAINS & PRODUCTS	.		.	.
485	Arrowroot, powder, dry		0.0	Swain 1985	
487	Barley, unpearled, dry		0.0	Swain 1985	Sharon 2007
489	Buckwheat, grains, dry	Schmutz2006	0.0	Swain 1985	
492	Maize, meal, dry		4.3	Swain 1985	Sharon

No	Name	Mast cell degranulators	Salicylates	Reference Salicylates	Lectin activity
					2007
494	Millet, grains, dry		0.0	Swain 1985	
495	Millet, hulled grains, dry		0.0	Swain 1985	
497	Oats, meal, dry		0.0	Swain 1985	Sharon 2007
500	Rice, brown grains, dry		0.0	Swain 1985	Sharon 2007
501	Rice, white grains, dry		0.0	Swain 1985	Sharon 2007
503	Rye, rolled, dry		0.0	Swain 1985	Sharon 2007
507	Sweet corn, fresh		1.3	Swain 1985	
508	Sweet corn, Mountain Maid creamed, canned		3.9	Swain 1985	
509	Sweet corn, Mountain Maid niblets, canned		2.6	Swain 1985	
513	Wheat, grains, dry		0.0	Swain 1985	Sharon 2007
514	**FRUIT & PRODUCTS**	.			.
516	Apple, Ardmona, canned		5.5	Swain 1985	Sharon 2007
517	Apple, Golden Delicious, fresh		0.8	Swain 1985	Sharon 2007
518	Apple, Granny Smith, fresh		5.9	Swain 1985	Sharon 2007
519	Apple, Jonathan, fresh		3.8	Swain 1985	Sharon 2007
520	Apple, Mountain Maid, juice		1.9	Swain 1985	Sharon 2007
521	Apple, Red Delicious, fresh		1.9	Swain 1985	Sharon 2007
522	Apricot, Ardmona, canned		14.2	Swain 1985	
523	Apricot, fresh		25.8	Swain 1985	
524	Apricot, Letona, nectar		1.4	Swain 1985	
526	Avocado, fresh		6.0	Swain 1985	
528	Banana, fresh		0.0	Swain 1985	Sharon 2007
530	Blackberry, John West, canned		18.6	Swain 1985	Sharon 2007
531	Blueberry, Socomin, canned		27.6	Swain 1985	
532	Boysenberry, John West, canned		20.4	Swain 1985	
534	Canteloupe, Australian rockmelon, fresh		15.0	Swain 1985	Sharon 2007
536	Cherry, John West, canned		27.8	Swain 1985	Sharon 2007
537	Cherry, Morello Sour, canned		3.0	Swain 1985	Sharon 2007
538	Cherry, sweet, fresh		8.5	Swain 1985	Sharon 2007
539	Cranberry, S. & W., canned		16.4	Swain 1985	
540	Cranberry, sauce		14.4	Swain 1985	
542	Currants, black currant, frozen		30.6	Swain 1985	Sharon 2007
543	Currants, red currant, frozen		50.6	Swain 1985	Sharon 2007

No	Name	Mast cell degranulators	Salicylates	Reference Salicylates	Lectin activity
544	Custard apple, (from Quensland), fresh		2.1	Swain 1985	
546	Dates, Cal-Date, dried		45.0	Swain 1985	
547	Dates, fresh		37.3	Swain 1985	
549	Figs, Calamata string, dried		6.4	Swain 1985	
550	Figs, fresh		1.8	Swain 1985	
551	Figs, S. & W. Kadota, canned		2.5	Swain 1985	
553	Grapefruit, Berri, juice	Maintz2007, Schmutz2006	4.2	Swain 1985	Sharon 2007
554	Grapefruit, fresh	Maintz2007, Schmutz2006	6.8	Swain 1985	Sharon 2007
556	Grapes, Berri Dark, juice		8.8	Swain 1985	
557	Grapes, currants I.P.C., dried		58.0	Swain 1985	
558	Grapes, raisins A.D.F.A., dried		66.2	Swain 1985	
559	Grapes, Red Malaita, fresh		9.4	Swain 1985	
560	Grapes, S. & W. light seedless, canned		1.6	Swain 1985	
561	Grapes, Sanitarium Light, juice		1.8	Swain 1985	
562	Grapes, sultana, dried		78.0	Swain 1985	
563	Grapes, Sultana, fresh		18.8	Swain 1985	
564	Guava, Gold Reef, canned		20.2	Swain 1985	
567	Kiwi fruit, fresh		3.2	Swain 1985	
570	Lemon, fresh	Vlieg2005, Schmutz2006, Maintz2007	1.8	Swain 1985	Sharon 2007
571	Logonberry, John West, canned		44.0	Swain 1985	
572	Loquat, fresh		2.6	Swain 1985	
573	Lychee, canned		3.6	Swain 1985	
575	Mandarin, fresh	Schmutz2006	5.6	Swain 1985	Sharon 2007
577	Mango, fresh	Schmutz2006	1.1	Swain 1985	
578	Watermelon				Sharon 2007
579	Mulberry, fresh		7.6	Swain 1985	
580	Nectarine, fresh		4.9	Swain 1985	
582	Orange, Berri, juice	Maintz2007, Schmutz2006	1.8	Swain 1985	Sharon 2007
583	Orange, fresh	Maintz2007, Schmutz2006	23.9	Swain 1985	Sharon 2007
584	Papaya	Vlieg2005, Schmutz2006, Maintz2007			Sharon 2007
586	Passion fruit, fresh		1.4	Swain 1985	
587	Pawpaw, fresh		0.8	Swain 1985	
588	Peach, fresh		5.8	Swain 1985	
589	Peach, Letona, canned		6.8	Swain 1985	
590	Peach, Letona, nectar		1.0	Swain 1985	
592	Pear, Letona Bartlett, canned		0.0	Swain 1985	
593	Pear, Packham (no skin), fresh		0.0	Swain 1985	

No	Name	Mast cell degranulators	Salicylates	Reference Salicylates	Lectin activity
594	Pear, Packham (with skin), fresh		2.7	Swain 1985	
595	Pear, William (with skin), fresh		3.1	Swain 1985	
596	Persimmon, fresh		1.8	Swain 1985	
598	Pineapple, fresh	Vlieg2005, Schmutz2006, Maintz2007	21.0	Swain 1985	
599	Pineapple, Golden Circle, canned	Vlieg2005, Schmutz2006, Maintz2007	13.6	Swain 1985	
600	Pineapple, Golden Circle, juice	Vlieg2005, Schmutz2006, Maintz2007	1.6	Swain 1985	
601	Plum, Blood (red), fresh		2.1	Swain 1985	Sharon 2007
603	Plum, Kelsey (green), fresh		1.0	Swain 1985	Sharon 2007
604	Plum, Letona prunes, canned		68.7	Swain 1985	Sharon 2007
605	Plum, S.P.C. dark red, canned		11.6	Swain 1985	Sharon 2007
606	Plum, Wilson (red), fresh		1.1	Swain 1985	Sharon 2007
607	Pomegranate				Sharon 2007
608	Pomegranate, fresh		0.7	Swain 1985	
610	Raspberries, fresh		31.4	Swain 1985	Sharon 2007
611	Raspberries, frozen		38.8	Swain 1985	Sharon 2007
614	Rhubarb, fresh		1.3	Swain 1985	
616	Strawberry, fresh	Vlieg2005, Schmutz2006, Maintz2007	13.6	Swain 1985	Sharon 2007
617	Tamarillo, fresh		1.0	Swain 1985	
618	Tangelo, fresh		7.2	Swain 1985	
619	Watermelon, fresh		4.8	Swain 1985	Sharon 2007
620	Youngberry, canned		30.6	Swain 1985	
621	**DRINKS**				
622	"Aktavite", powder		0.0	Swain 1985	
623	"Milo", powder		0.1	Swain 1985	
624	"Ovaltine", powder		0.0	Swain 1985	
625	Cereal coffee, "Ecco", powder		0.0	Swain 1985	
626	Cereal coffee, "Nature's Cuppa", powder		22.6	Swain 1985	
627	Cereal coffee, "Reform", powder		3.8	Swain 1985	
628	Cereal coffee, Bambu, powder		1.5	Swain 1985	
629	Cereal coffee, Dandelion, powder		0.8	Swain 1985	
630	Coca-cola, liquid		2.5	Swain 1985	
632	Coffee, Andronicus Instant, powder		0.0	Swain 1985	Sharon 2007
633	Coffee, Bushells Instant, powder		2.1	Swain 1985	Sharon 2007

No	Name	Mast cell degranulators	Salicylates	Reference Salicylates	Lectin activity
634	Coffee, Bushells Turkish Style, powder		1.9	Swain 1985	Sharon 2007
635	Coffee, Gibsons Instant, powder		1.2	Swain 1985	Sharon 2007
636	Coffee, Harris Instant I, powder		0.0	Swain 1985	Sharon 2007
637	Coffee, Harris Instant II, powder		1.0	Swain 1985	Sharon 2007
638	Coffee, Harris Mocha Kenya, beans		4.5	Swain 1985	Sharon 2007
639	Coffee, International Roast, powder		9.6	Swain 1985	Sharon 2007
640	Coffee, Maxwell House Instant, powder		8.4	Swain 1985	Sharon 2007
641	Coffee, Moccona Decaffeinated, powder		0.0	Swain 1985	Sharon 2007
642	Coffee, Moccona Instant, granules		6.4	Swain 1985	Sharon 2007
643	Coffee, Nescafe Decaffeinated, powder		0.0	Swain 1985	Sharon 2007
644	Coffee, Nescafe Instant, granules		5.9	Swain 1985	Sharon 2007
645	Coffee, Robert Timms Instant, powder		0.0	Swain 1985	Sharon 2007
646	Rose hip, Delrose, syrup	EC 2012: contact allergen	11.7	Swain 1985	
647	Tea, Asco, bag		64.0	Swain 1985	
648	Tea, Billy, leaves		24.8	Swain 1985	
649	Tea, Burmese Green, leaves		29.7	Swain 1985	
650	Tea, Bushells, bag		47.8	Swain 1985	
651	Tea, camomille, bag		0.6	Swain 1985	
653	Tea, fruit, bag		3.6	Swain 1985	
654	Tea, Goldon Days Decaffeinated, bag		3.7	Swain 1985	
655	Tea, Harris, bag		40.0	Swain 1985	
656	Tea, Indian Green, leaves		29.7	Swain 1985	
659	Tea, Old Chinese, leaves		19.0	Swain 1985	
660	Tea, Peony Jasmine, leaves		19.0	Swain 1985	
662	Tea, peppermint, bag	EC 2012: contact allergen	11.0	Swain 1985	
664	Tea, rose hip, bag	EC 2012: contact allergen	4.0	Swain 1985	
665	Tea, Tetley, bag		55.7	Swain 1985	
666	Tea, Twinings - Darjeeling, leaves		42.4	Swain 1985	
667	Tea, Twinings - Earl Grey, bag	EC 2012: contact allergen	30.0	Swain 1985	
668	Tea, Twinings - English Breakfast, bag		30.0	Swain 1985	
669	Tea, Twinings - Irish Breakfast, bag		38.9	Swain 1985	
670	Tea, Twinings - Lapsang Souchong, bag		24.0	Swain 1985	
671	Tea, Twinings - Lemon Scented, bag	EC 2012: contact allergen	73.4	Swain 1985	

No	Name	Mast cell degranulators	Salicylates	Reference Salicylates	Lectin activity
672	Tea, Twinings - Orange Pekoe, leaves	EC 2012: contact allergen	27.5	Swain 1985	
673	Tea, Twinings - Prince of Wales, bag		29.7	Swain 1985	
674	ALCOHOLIC DRINKS				
683	Beer, Reschs Dinner Ale	Intorre1996	3.5	Swain 1985	
684	Beer, Tooheys Draught	Intorre1996	2.3	Swain 1985	
685	Beer, Tooths Sheaf Stout	Intorre1996	3.2	Swain 1985	
688	Cider, Bulmer's Dry		1.7	Swain 1985	
689	Cider, Bulmer's Sweet		1.9	Swain 1985	
690	Cider, Lilydale Dry		1.7	Swain 1985	
691	Cider, Mercury Dry		1.6	Swain 1985	
694	Liqueurs, Benedictine		90.4	Swain 1985	
695	Liqueurs, Cointreau		6.6	Swain 1985	
696	Liqueurs, Drambui		16.8	Swain 1985	
697	Liqueurs, Tia Maria		8.3	Swain 1985	
698	Port, McWilliams Royal Reserve		14.0	Swain 1985	
699	Port, Stonyfell Mellow		42.0	Swain 1985	
701	Sherry, Lindemans Royal Reserve Sweet		5.6	Swain 1985	
702	Sherry, Mildara Supreme Dry		4.6	Swain 1985	
703	Sherry, Penfolds Royal Reserve Sweet		4.9	Swain 1985	
704	Spirits, brandy-Hennessy		4.0	Swain 1985	
705	Spirits, gin-Gilbey's		0.0	Swain 1985	
706	Spirits, rum-Bundaberg		7.6	Swain 1985	
707	Spirits, rum-Captain Morgan		12.8	Swain 1985	
708	Spirits, vodka-Smirnoff		0.0	Swain 1985	
709	Spirits, whiskey-Johnnie Walker		0.0	Swain 1985	
721	Wines, Buton Dry Vermouth		4.6	Swain 1985	
722	Wines, Kaiser Stuhl Rose		3.7	Swain 1985	
723	Wines, Lindemans Riesling		8.1	Swain 1985	
724	Wines, McWilliams Cabernet Sauvignon		8.6	Swain 1985	
725	Wines, McWilliams Dry White Wine		1.0	Swain 1985	
726	Wines, McWilliams Private Bin Claret		9.0	Swain 1985	
727	Wines, McWilliams Reserve Claret		3.5	Swain 1985	
728	Wines, Penfolds Traminer Riesling Bin 202		8.1	Swain 1985	
729	Wines, Seaview Rhine Riesling		8.9	Swain 1985	
730	Wines, Stonyfell Ma Chere		6.9	Swain 1985	
731	Wines, Yalumba Champagne		10.2	Swain 1985	
732	SUGAR & SWEETS				

No	Name	Mast cell degranulators	Salicylates	Reference Salicylates	Lectin activity
733	Caramel, Pascall Cream, dry		1.2	Swain 1985	
734	Carob, powder, dry		0.0	Swain 1985	
740	Cocoa, powder, dry		0.0	Swain 1985	Sharon 2007
741	Golden syrup, C.S.R., liquid		1.0	Swain 1985	
743	Honey, "No Frills", liquid		112.4	Swain 1985	
744	Honey, Allowire, liquid		25.0	Swain 1985	
745	Honey, Aristocrat, liquid		37.0	Swain 1985	
746	Honey, Capillano, liquid		101.4	Swain 1985	
747	Honey, Mudgee, liquid		39.0	Swain 1985	
748	Licorice, Barratts, dry		97.8	Swain 1985	
749	Licorice, Giant, dry		79.6	Swain 1985	
750	Maple syrup, Camp, liquid		0.0	Swain 1985	
751	Molasses, C.S.R., liquid		2.2	Swain 1985	
752	Peppermints, "Mintiers", dry		17.8	Swain 1985	
753	Peppermints, Allens "Koolmint", dry		75.8	Swain 1985	
754	Peppermints, Allens "Steamrollers", dry		29.2	Swain 1985	
755	Peppermints, Allens Strong Mint, dry		7.7	Swain 1985	
756	Peppermints, Lifesavers, dry		8.6	Swain 1985	
757	Sugar, white granulated, dry		0.0	Swain 1985	
758	CONDIMENTS (SPICES, HERBS, SAUCES)	.		.	.
759	"Bonox", liquid		2.8	Swain 1985	
760	"Marmite", Sanitarium, paste		7.1	Swain 1985	
761	"Vegemite", Kraft, paste		8.1	Swain 1985	
763	Allspice, powder, dry		52.0	Swain 1985	Sharon 2007
764	Aniseed, powder, dry		228.0	Swain 1985	
765	Asafoetida		38.0	Paterson 2006	
766	Basil, powder, dry		34.0	Swain 1985	
768	Bay leaf, leaves, dry	EC 2012: contact allergen	25.2	Swain 1985	
770	Canella, powder, dry		426.0	Swain 1985	
772	Caraway, powder, dry		28.2	Swain 1985	Sharon 2007
773	Cardamom, black		270.0	Paterson 2006	
774	Cardamom, green		132.0	Paterson 2006	
775	Cardamom, powder, dry		77.0	Swain 1985	
776	Cayenne, powder, dry		176.0	Swain 1985	
777	Celery, powder, dry		101.0	Swain 1985	
778	Chili, flakes, dry		13.8	Swain 1985	
779	Chili, powder, dry		13.0	Swain 1985	
780	Chilli, red powder		1466.0	Paterson 2006	
782	Cinnamon	EC 2012: contact allergen	642.0	Paterson 2006	

No	Name	Mast cell degranulators	Salicylates	Reference Salicylates	Lectin activity
783	Cinnamon, powder, dry	EC 2012: contact allergen	152.0	Swain 1985	
785	Cloves	EC 2012: contact allergen	25.0	Paterson 2006	
786	Cloves, whole, dry	EC 2012: contact allergen	57.4	Swain 1985	
787	Coriander		27.0	Paterson 2006	
788	Coriander, leaves, fresh		2.0	Swain 1985	
789	Cumin		16294.0	Paterson 2006	
790	Cumin, powder, dry		450.0	Swain 1985	
791	Curry, powder, dry		2180.0	Swain 1985	
792	Dill, fresh		69.0	Swain 1985	
793	Dill, powder, dry		944.0	Swain 1985	
794	Fennel		20.0	Paterson 2006	
795	Fennel, powder, dry		8.0	Swain 1985	
796	Fenugreek		1.0	Paterson 2006	
797	Fenugreek, powder, dry		122.0	Swain 1985	
798	Five spice, powder, dry		308.0	Swain 1985	
799	Garam masala, powder, dry		668.0	Swain 1985	
800	Garlic		56.0	Paterson 2006	
801	Garlic, bulbs, fresh		1.0	Swain 1985	
802	Ginger		35.0	Paterson 2006	
803	Ginger, root, fresh		45.0	Swain 1985	
805	Mace, powder, dry		322.0	Swain 1985	
806	Marjoram				Sharon 2007
807	Mint, common garden, fresh		94.0	Swain 1985	Sharon 2007
808	Mixed herbs, leaves, dry		556.0	Swain 1985	
810	Mustard	Schmutz2006	262.0	Paterson 2006	
811	Mustard, powder, dry	Schmutz2006	260.0	Swain 1985	
813	Nutmeg, powder, dry		24.0	Swain 1985	Sharon 2007
814	Oregano, powder, dry		660.0	Swain 1985	
815	Paprika		1043.0	Paterson 2006	
816	Paprika, hot powder, dry		2030.0	Swain 1985	
817	Paprika, sweet powder, dry		57.0	Swain 1985	
819	Parsley, leaves, fresh		0.8	Swain 1985	Sharon 2007
820	Pepper, black powder, dry		62.0	Swain 1985	
821	Pepper, black seeds		90.0	Paterson 2006	
822	Pepper, white powder, dry		11.0	Swain 1985	
823	Peppermint	EC 2012: contact allergen			Sharon 2007
824	Pimiento, powder, dry		49.0	Swain 1985	
825	Rosemary, powder, dry		680.0	Swain 1985	
826	Saffron, powder, dry		0.0	Swain 1985	

No	Name	Mast cell degranulators	Salicylates	Reference Salicylates	Lectin activity
827	Sage, leaves, dry		217.0	Swain 1985	
828	Soy sauce, liquid		0.0	Swain 1985	
829	Tabasco pepper, Mcilhenny, sauce		4.5	Swain 1985	
830	Tamarind		96.0	Paterson 2006	
831	Tandori, powder, dry		0.0	Swain 1985	
832	Tarragon, powder, dry		348.0	Swain 1985	
833	Thyme, leaves, dry		1830.0	Swain 1985	
834	Turmeric		3505.0	Paterson 2006	
835	Turmeric, powder, dry		764.0	Swain 1985	
836	Vanilla, essence, liquid		14.4	Swain 1985	
839	Vinegar, malt, liquid	Schmutz2006	0.0	Swain 1985	
841	Vinegar, white, liquid	Schmutz2006	13.3	Swain 1985	
842	Worcestershire sauce, liquid		643.0	Swain 1985	

References for food list tables

- Databank voor voedselovergevoeligheid ALBA, Zeist (1996) Biogene aminen in voedingsmiddelen
- Ansorena D, Montelb MC, Rokkac M, Tolonb R, Eerolac S, Rizzoc A, Raemaekersd M, Demeyerd D (2002) Analysis of biogenic amines in northern and southern European sausages and role of flora in amine production, Meat Sci. 61: 141-147
- Bardócz S. et al. (1993) Polyamines in food - implications for growth and health, J. Nutr. Biochem. 4: 66
- Bover-Cid S, Izquierdo-Pulido M, Vidal-Carou MC (1999) Effect of proteolytic starter cultures of Staphylococcus spp. on biogenic amine formation during ripening of dry fermented sausages, Int. J. Food Microbiol. 46: 95-104
- Bover-Cid S, Schoppen S, Izquierdo-Pulido M, Vidal-Carou MC (1999) Relationship between biogenic amine contents and the size of dry fermented sausages, Meat Sci. 51: 305-311
- Coïsson JD et al. (2004) Production of biogenic amines in "Salamini italiani alla cacciatora PDO", Meat Science 67/2: 343-349
- Coïsson JD, Travaglia F, Barile D, Cereti E, Arlorio M (2008) Determination of biogenic amines in Parmesan grated cheese samples, 5th IDF Symposiumon Cheese Ripening
- De Borba BM, Rohrer JS (2007) Determination of biogenic amines in alcoholic beverages by ion chromatography with suppressed conductivity detection and integrated pulsed amperometric detection, J. Chromatogr. A 1155: 22-30
- Den Brinker C et al. (1995) Investigation of biogenic amines in fish and fish products, Victorian Government Department of Human Services
- Dionex (2007) Determination of biogenic amines in fruit, vegetables, and chocolate using ion chromatography with suppressed conductivity and integrated pulsed amperometric detections; Application Update 162, 8 pages
- Eerola S, Maijala R, Roig Sagués AX, Salminen M, Hirvi T (1996) Biogenic amines in dry sausages as affected by starter culture and contaminant amine-positive Lactobacillus, J. Food Sci. 61: 1243-1246
- Eerola HS, Roig Sagués AX, Hirvi TK (1998) Biogenic amines in Finnish dry sausages, J. Food Saf. 18: 127-138
- EFSA (2004) Opinion of the Scientific Panel on Dietetic Products, Nutrition and Allergies on a request from the Commission relating to the evaluation of allergenic foods for labelling purposes, EFSA Journal (2004) 32, 1-197
- EFSA (2010) Scientific Opinion on the appropriateness of the food azo-colours Tartrazine (E 102), Sunset Yellow FCF (E 110), Carmoisine (E 122), Amaranth (E 123), Ponceau 4R (E 124), Allura Red AC (E 129), Brilliant Black BN (E 151), Brown FK (E 154), Brown HT (E 155) and Litholrubine BK (E 180) for inclusion in the list of food ingredients set up in Annex IIIa of Directive 2000/13/EC, EFSA Journal 2010;8(10):1778
- El-Sayed MM (1996) Biogenic amines in processed cheese available in Egypt, Int. Dairy J. 6: 1079
- Emborg J, Dalgaard P (2006) Formation of histamine nad biogenic amines in cold-smoked tuna: an investigation of psychrotolerant bacteria from samples implicated in cases of histamine fish poisoning, J. Food Prot. 69: 897-906
- Ferreira V, et al. (2006) Chemical and microbiological characterization of alheira: A typical Portuguese fermented sausage with particular reference to factors relating to food safety, Meat Science 73/4: 570-575
- Ferreira V, Barbosa J, Silva J, Vendeiro S, Mota A, Siva F, Monteiro MJ, Hogg T, Gibbs P, Teixeira P (2007) Chemical and microbiological characterization of "Salpicão de Vinhais" and "Chouriça de Vinhais": traditional dry sausages produced in the north of Portugal, Food Microbiol. 24: 618-623
- Garai G, Duenas MT, Irastorza A, Martin-Alvarez PJ, Moreno-Arribas MV (2006) Biogenic amines in natural ciders, J. Food Prot. 69: 3006-3012
- Genccelep H, Kaban G, Kaya M (2007) Effects of starter cultures and nitrite levels on formation of biogenic amines in sucuk, Meat Sci. 77: 424-430
- Gil-Agusti M, Carda-Broch S, Monferrer-Pons L, Esteve-Romero J (2007) Simultaneous determination of tyramine and tryptamine and their precursor amino acids by micellar liquid chromatography and pulsed amperometric detection in wines, J. Chromatogr. A 1156: 288-295
- Gloria MBA, Izquierdo-Pulido M (1999) Levels and significance of biogenic amines in Brazilian beers, J. Food Composition Anal. 12: 129-136
- Gosetti F, Mazzucco E, Gianotti V, Polati S, Gennaro MC (2007) High performance liquid chromatography/tandem mass spectroscopy determination of biogenic amines in typical Piedmont cheeses, J. Chromatogr. A 1149: 151-157
- Hernandez-Jover T, Izquierdo-Pulido M, Veciana-Nogues MT, Marine-Font A, Vidal-Carou MC (1997) Biogenic amine and polyamine contents in meat and meat products, J. Agric. Food Chem. 45: 2098-2102
- Ibrahim EMA, Amer AA (2010) Comparison of biogenic amines levels in different processed cheese varieties with regulatory specifications, World Journal of Dairy & Food Sciences 5/2, 127-133
- Innocente N, Dagostin P (2002) Formation of biogenic amines in a typical semihard Italian cheese, J. Food Prot. 65: 1498

- Intorre L, Bertini S, Luchetti E, Mengozzi G, Crema F, Soldami G (1996) The effect of ethanol, beer, and wine on histamine release from the dog stomach, Alcohol, 13/6: 547-551
- Izquierdo P, Allara M, Torres G, García A, Barboza Y , Isabel Piñero M (2003) Revista Científica, FCV-LUZ / Vol. XIII, Nº 6, 431-435, 431-435
- Komprda T, Neznalova J, Standara S, Bover-Cid S (2001) Effect of starter culture and storage temperature on the content of biogenic amines in dry fermented sausages Poličane, Meat Sci. 59: 267-276
- Komprda T, Smela D, Pechova P, Kalhotka L, Stencl J, Klejdus B (2004) Effect of starter culture, spice mix and storage time and temperature on biogenic amine content of dry fermented sausages, Meat Sci. 67: 607-616
- Komprda T, et al. (2005) Biogenic amine content in sterilized and pasteurized long-term stored processed cheese, Czech J. Food Sci. 23: 209
- Komprda T, et al. (2007) Content and distribution of biogenic amines in Dutch-type hard cheese, Food Chem. 102: 129
- Komprda T, et al. (2008) Biogenic amine and polyamine contents in a Czech blue-vein cheese, Czech J. Food Sci 26/6: 428-440
- Komprda T, et al. (2008) Some factors influencing biogenic amines and polyamines contents in Dutch-type semi-hard cheese, Eur. Food Res. Technol. 227: 29
- Komprda T, Dohnal V (2010 in press) Chapter 41 Amines, pages 865-882, In: L.M. Nollet, F. Toldra (editors) Handbook of Dairy Food Analysis, CRS Press, Taylor and Francis
- Konakovsky V, Focke M, Hoffmann-Sommergruber K, Schmid R, Scheiner O, Moser P, Jarisch R, Hemmer W (2011) Levels of histamine and other biogenic amines in high-quality red wines, Addit Contam Part A Chem Anal Control Expo Risk Assess Feb 16: 1-9
- Koutsoumanis K, Tassou C, Nychas GJE (2010) Biogenic amines in foods (Chapter 16), In: Pathogens and Toxins in Foods: Challenges and Interventions, ed. VK Juneja, JN Sofos, ASM Press, Washington DC
- Kung HF, Lee YH, Chang SC, Wei CI, Tsai YH (2007) Histamine contents and histamine-forming bacteria in sufu products in Taiwan, Food Control 18: 381-386
- Kung HF, Tsai YH, Wei CI (2007) Histamine and other biogenic amines and histamine-forming bacteria in miso products, Food Chem. 101: 351-356
- Ladero V, et al. (2011) Biogenic amines content in Spanish and French natural ciders: Application of qPCR for quantitative detection of biogenic amine-producers, Food Microbiology 28(3): 554-61
- Latorre-Moratalla ML, Veciana-Nogués T, Bover-Cid S, Garriga M, Aymerich T, Zanardi E, Ianieri A, Fraqueza MJ, Patarata L, . Drosinos EH, Lauková A, Talon R, Vidal-Carou MC (2008) Biogenic amines in traditional fermented sausages produced in selected European countries, Food Chemistry, 107/2, 912–921
- Lauryssen S, Nauwelaers I (2005) Ongewenste gast op ons bord, TEST GEZONDHEID 67: 9-11
- Leuscher RGK, Kurihara R, Hammes WP (1998) Effect of enhanced proteolysis on formation of biogenic amines by lactobacilli during Gouda cheese ripening, Int. J. Food Microbiol. 44: 15
- Lu Yongmeia, Chen Xiaohonga, Jiang Meia, Lv Xina, Nurgul Rahmanb, Dong Mingshenga, and Gujun Yanc (2009) Biogenic amines in Chinese soy sauce, Food Control 20/6: 593-597
- Marcobal A, et al. (2005) Biogenic amine content of red Spanish wines: comparison of a direct ELISA and an HPLC method for the determination of histamine in   wines,   Food Research International 38/4: 387-394
- Marino M, Maifreni M, Moret S, Rondinini G (2000) The capacity of Enterobacteriaceae species to produce biogenic amines in cheese, Lett. Appl. Microbiol. 31: 169-173
- Mendes R (1999) Changes in biogenic amines of major Portugese bluefish species during storage at different temperatures, J. Food Biochem 23/1: 33-43
- Montel MC, Masson F, Talon R (1999) Comparison of biogenic amine content in traditional and industrial French dry sausages, Sci. Aliments 19: 247-254
- Mendes R, Goncalves A, Nunes ML (1999) Changes in free amino acids and biogenic amines during ripening of fresh and frozen sardines, J. Food Biochem 23/3: 295-306
- Nishino N, Hattori H, Wada H, Touno E (2007) Biogenic amine production in grass, maize and total mixed ration silages inoculated with Lactobacillus casei or Lactobacillus buchneri, J. Appl Microbiol. 103(2): 325-332
- Novella-Rodrígues S, et al. (2000) Biogenic amines and polyamines in milks and cheeses by ion-pair high performance liquid chromatography, J. Agric. Food Chem. 48: 5117
- Novella-Rodrígues S, et al. (2002) Influence of starter and nonstarter on the formation of biogenic amine in goat cheese during ripening, J. Dairy Sci. 85: 2471
- Novella- Rodrígues S, Veciana-Nogues MT, Izquierdo-Pulido M, Vidal-Carou MC (2003) Distribution of biogenic amines and polyamines in cheese, J. Food Sci. 68: 750-755
- Novella-Rodrígues S, et al. (2004) Evaluation of biogenic amines and microbial counts throughout the ripening of goat cheeses from pasteurized and raw milk, J. Dairy Res. 71: 245
- Özogul F, Özogul Y (2006) Biogenic amine content and biogenic amine quality indices of sardines (Sardina pilchardus) stored in modified atmosphere packaging and vacuum packaging, Food Chem. 99: 574-578

- Parente E, Martuscelli M, Gardini F, Grieco S, Crudele MA, Suzzi G (2001) Evolution of microbial populations and biogenic amine production in dry sausages produced in Southern Italy, J. Appl. Microbiol. 90: 882-891
- Petridis KD, Steinhart H (1999) Biogene amine in der Hartkäseproduktion: I. Einfluss verschiedener Parameter auf den Amingehalt im Endprodukt am Beispiel von Emmentaler Käse, Deutsche Lebensmittel-Rundschau 92: 114
- Pinho O, et al. (2001) Effect of temperature on evolution of free amino acid and biogenic amine contents during storage of Azeitão cheese, Food Chem. 75: 287
- Pinho O, et al. (2004) Interrelationships among microbiological, physicochemical, and biochemical properties of Terrincho cheese, with emphasis on biogenic amines, J. Food Prot. 67: 2779
- Pons-Sanchez-Cascado S, Veciana-Nogues MT, Bover-Cid S, Marine-Font A, Vidal-Carou MC (2005) Volatile and biogenic amines, microbiological counts, and bacterial amino acid decarboxylase activity throughout the salt-ripening process of anchovies (Engraulis encrasicholus), J Food Prot. 68: 1683-1689
- Rabie MA, Elsaidy A, El-Badawy AA, Siliha H, Malcata FX (2011) Biogenic Amine Contents in Selected Egyptian Fermented Foods as Determined by Ion-Exchange Chromatography, J Food Prot. 74(4): 681-685
- Rezaei M, Montazeri N, Langrudi, HE, Mokhayer M, Parviz M, Nazarinia 2007 (2007) The biogenic amines and bacterial changes of farmed rainbow trout (Oncorhynchus mykiss) stored in ice, Food Chem 103: 150-154
- Roig-Sagués AX, Molina AP, Hernándes-Herrero MM (2002) Histamine and tyramine-forming microorganisms in Spanish traditional cheeses, Eur. Food Res. Technol. 215: 96
- Roseiro C, Santos C, Sol M, Silva L, Fernandes I (2006) Prevalence of biogenic amines during ripening of a traditional dry fermented pork sausage and its relation to the amount of sodium chloride added, Meat Sci 74: 557-563
- Ruiz-Capillas C, Moral A (2001) Effect of controlled atmospheres enriched in O2 in formation of biogenic amines in chilled hake (Merluccius merluccius L.), Eur Food Res Technol 212: 546-550
- Ruiz-Capillas C, Moral A (2001) Formation of biogenic amines in bulk-stored chilled hake (Merluccius merluccius L) packed under atmospheres, Journal of Food Protection 64/7: 1045-1050
- Ruiz-Capillas C, Moral A (2001) Production of biogenic amines and their potential use as quality control indices for hake (Merluccius merluccius L.) stored in ice, Journal of Food Science 66/7: 1030-1032
- Ruiz-Capillas C, Jiménez-Colmenero F (2004) Biogenic amine content in Spanish retail market meat products treated with protective atmosphere and high pressure, Eur Food Res Technol 218: 237-241
- Ruiz-Capillas C, Moral A (2004) Free amino acids and biogenic amines in red and white muscle of tuna stored in controlled atmospheres, Amino Acids 26: 125-132
- Ruiz-Capillas C, Carballo J, Jimenez Colmenero F (2007) Biogenic amines in pressurized vacuum-packaged cooked sliced ham under different chilled storage conditions, Meat Sci. 75: 397-405
- Santamaria P (2006) Nitrate in vegetables: toxicity, content, intake and EC regulation. Review, J.Sci.Food Agric. 86: 10-17
- Schirone M, Tofalo R, Mazzone G, Corsetti A, Suzzi G (2011) Biogenic amine content and microbiological profile of Pecorino de Farindola cheese, Food Microbiology 28: 128-136
- Schneller R, Good P, Jenney M (1997) Influence of pasteurised milk, raw milk, and different ripening cultures on biogenic amine concentrations in semi-soft cheeses during ripening, Z. Lebensm. Untersuch. Forsch. A 204: 265
- Shalaby AR (1993) Survey on biogenic amines in Egyptian foods: sausages, J. Sci. Food Agric. 62: 219-224
- Sharon N, Lis H (2007) Lectins, 2nd edition, Springer, ISBN 978-1-4020-6605-4 paperback, 454 pages
- Simon-Sarkadi L, Holzapfel WH, Halasz A (1994) Biogenic amine content and microbial contamination of leafy vegetables during storage at 5°C, J. Food Biochem. 17: 407-418
- Ten Brink B, Damink C, Joosten HMLJ, Juis in 't Veld JHJ (1990) Occurence and formation of biologically active amines in foods, Int. J. Food Microbiol. 11: 73-84
- Tsai YH, Kung HF, Lee TM, Chen HC, Chou SS, Wei CI, Hwang DF (2005) Determination of histamine in canned mackerel implicated in a food borne poisoning, Food Control 16: 579-585
- Tsai YH, Lin CY, Chang SC, Chenc HC, Kung HF, Wei CI, Hwang DF (2005) Occurrence of histamine and histamine-forming bacteria in salted mackerel in Taiwan, Food Microbiol. 22: 461-467
- Tsai YH, et al. (2006) Histamine content of fermented fish products in Taiwan and isolation of histamine-forming bacteria, Food Chemistry, 98/1: 64-70
- Tsai YH, Chang SC, Kung HF (2007) Histamine contents and histamine-forming bacteria in natto products in Taiwan, Food Control 18: 1026-1030
- Valsamaki K, Michaelidou A, Polychroniadou A (2000) Biogenic amine production in Feta cheese, Food Chem. 71: 259
- Vandekerckhove P (1977) Amines in dry fermented sausages, J. Food Sci. 42: 283-285

- Veciana-Nogués MT, Mariné Font A, Vidal Carou MC (1997) Biogenic amines as hygienic quality indicators of tuna. Relationships with microbial counts, ATP-related compounds, volatile and organoleptic changes, J Agric Food Chem 45/6: 2036-2041
- Vinci G, Antonelli ML (2002) Biogenic amines: quality index of freshness in red and white meat, Food Control 13: 519-524
- Virgili R, Saccani G, Gabba L, Tanzi E, Soresi Bordini C (2007) Changes of free amino acids and biogenic amines during extended ageing of Italian dry-cured ham, Lebensm. Wiss. Technol. 40: 871-878
- Vlieg-Boerstra BJ, et al. (2005) Mastocytosis and adverse reactions to biogenic amines and histamine-releasing foods: what is the evidence? Journal of Medicine 63/7: 244-249
- Yeh CY, et al. (2004) Biogenic amines and histamine of marlin fillet and spotted mackeral fillet sampled from cafeteria and anchovy from fish market in Keelung, Journal of Food and Drug Analysis, 12/2: 128-132

APPENDIX 3: REFERENCES

English books

Dirk Budka (unknown; purchased as pdf file July 2012) The Histamine Confusion, ISBN 978-0-9557205-2-9
- This book does not decrease the confusion.
- Medical terms are not explained.
- No in-text references provided.
- No food list.
- Are laser blood irradiation and low level laser therapy (LLLT) evidence based?
- Not independent because the author gives paid medical advice on this topic.

Genny Masterman (2011) What HIT me? Living with Histamine Intolerance: A guide to diagnosis and management of HIT - A patient's point of view, CreateSpace ISBN 978-1456365615
- Clear explanation to improve the understanding.
- Food items in the food list do not show typical histamine concentrations.
- No in-text references provided
- Independent

Helmut Schmutz (2006) Food Intolerance (Histamine Intolerance) ISBN 9783950228700 (paperback), Publisher HSC, Mauerback.
- Good historical overview.
- Clear explanations which improve the understanding.
- Less practical because of limited food list.
- Not independent because the author is the seller of DAO enzyme and DAO tests.

Yasmina Ykelenstam "The Low Histamine Chef" (2012) Low histamine on the go
Yasmina Ykelenstam "The Low Histamine Chef" (2012) The low histamine dessert book
- Great inspiring recipes, also if you have no histamine intolerance/mast cell activation!

Articles

Déficit de actividad funcional de DAO. Acumulación de histamina
Duelo A
Medicos y Medicinas no.24, 28-30

Opinion on fragrance allergens in cosmetic products
European Commission, Scientific Committee on Consumer Safety
European Commission 2012, SCCS/1459/11, 334 pages,
http://ec.europa.eu/health/scientific_committees/consumer_safety/docs/sccs_o_102.pdf

The effect of Helicobacter pylori eradication on migraine: a randomized, double blind, controlled trial
Faraji F, Zarinfar N, Zanjani AT, Morteza A
Pain Physician. 2012;15(6): 495-8
BACKGROUND: Recent studies have shown a positive correlation between Helicobacter pylori (H. pylori)infection and migraine headache.
OBJECTIVE: To study the impact of H. pylori eradication on migraine headache.
STUDY DESIGN: Double blind, randomized, controlled clinical trial.
SETTING: Sixty-four patients diagnosed with migraine-type headache were included in the study. The patients were randomly allocated into 2 groups: a treatment group that received migraine treatment and H.pylori eradication treatment, and a control group that received migraine treatment and a placebo in place of H. pylori eradication treatment.
METHODS: There were 25 women and 7 men in the treatment group and 22 women and 10 men in the control group. The MIDAS (Migraine Disability Assessment) questionnaire was used to assess the severity of symptoms, before and after treatment.
RESULT:There was no significant difference between treatment group patients and control group patients with respect to age (44.6 ± 8.8 vs. 43.8 ± 13.8), clinical symptoms and signs. In the beginning of the study, patients in the treatment group had a higher MIDAS compared to patients in the control group (28.87 ± 6.18 vs. 25.43 ± 7.13, P < 0.05). There was no significant difference between the treatment and control groups, with respect to the MIDAS, after treatment (20.09 ± 1.14 vs. 20.00 ± 1.150, P = 0.5). General linear model, repeated measures demonstrated that the reduction in the MIDAS score was more prominent in the treatment group (Mean Square 164.25, F: 2.02, P = 0.05).
LIMITATIONS: Short-term follow up.
CONCLUSION: H. pylori eradication may have a beneficial role on migraine headache. This shows the significance of H. pylori treatment in the management of migraine headache among Iranian patients.

Mast Cell Activation Syndrome: A Review
Frieri M, Patel R, Celestin J
Curr Allergy Asthma Rep. 2012 Nov 22
Mast cell activation syndrome (MCAS) is a condition with signs and symptoms involving the skin, gastrointestinal, cardiovascular, respiratory, and neurologic systems. It can be classified into primary, secondary, and idiopathic. Earlier proposed criteria for the diagnosis of MCAS included episodic symptoms consistent with mast cell mediator release affecting two or more organ systems with urticaria, angioedema, flushing, nausea, vomiting, diarrhea, abdominal cramping, hypotensive syncope or near syncope, tachycardia, wheezing, conjunctival injection, pruritus, and nasal stuffiness. Other criteria included a decrease in the frequency, severity, or resolution of symptoms with anti-mediator therapy including H(1) and H(2)histamine receptor antagonists, anti-leukotrienes, or mast cell stabilizers. Laboratory data that support the diagnosis include an increase of a validated urinary or serum marker of mast cell activation (MCA), namely the documentation of an increase of the marker above the patient's baseline value during symptomatic periods on more than two occasions, or baseline serum tryptase levels that are persistently above 15 ng/ml, or documentation of an increase of the tryptase level above baseline value on one occasion. Less specific assays are 24-h urine histamine metabolites, PGD(2) (Prostaglandin D(2)) or its metabolite, 11-β-prostaglandin F(2) alpha. A recent global definition, criteria, and classification include typical clinical symptoms, a substantial transient increase in serum total tryptase level or an increase in other mast cell derived mediators, such as histamine or PGD2 or their urinary metabolites, and a response of clinical symptoms to agents that attenuate the production or activities of mast cell mediators.

[Histamine intolerance and pseudoallergy--do they exist?]. [Article in Finnish]
Hannuksela M, Haahtela T.
Duodecim. 2012; 128(9): 952-7
Histamine intolerance (HIT) is a controversial syndrome, in which the body is believed to react to histamine released by certain foodstuffs. Symptoms include among other things headache, urticaria

and abdominal discomfort. Several fruits, nuts, spices and food additives have been regarded as pseudoallergens. Since there is no objective investigation to prove HIT, the diagnosis is based on symptoms. On the basis of literature, better clinical studies are needed. Because
the phenomenon remains unclear, use of the terms histamine intolerance and pseudoallergens is not recommended.

Histaminintoleranz (HIT) Mit gezielter Anamnese zur richtigen Diagnose
Kofler, L., Kofler, H.
Der Deutsche Dermatologe 2012/2: 99-102
Mit dem Krankheitsbild der Histaminunverträglichkeit ist man in der täglichen Praxis immer öfter konfrontiert. Die Patienten haben oft eine lange Reihe an Arztkonsultationen und Untersuchungen hinter sich. Zur sorgfältigen Diagnosestellung der Erkrankung ist auch der Ausschluss von Differenzial-diagnosen und die Untersuchung auf Komorbiditäten wichtig.

Involvement of human histamine N-methyltransferase gene polymorphisms in susceptibility to atopic dermatitis in Korean children
Lee HS, Kim SH, Kim KW, Baek JY, Park HS, Lee KE, Hong JY, Kim MN, Heo WI, Sohn MH, Kim KE
Allergy Asthma Immunol Res. 2012 January; 4(1): 31–36
PURPOSE: Histamine N-methyltransferase (HNMT) catalyzes one of two major histamine metabolic pathways. Histamine is a mediator of pruritus in atopic dermatitis (AD). The aim of this study was to evaluate the association between HNMT polymorphisms and AD in children.
METHODS: We genotyped 763 Korean children for allelic determinants at four polymorphic sites in the HNMT gene: -465T>C, -413C>T, 314C>T, and 939A>G. Genotyping was performed using a TaqMan fluorogenic 5' nuclease assay. The functional effect of the 939A>G polymorphism was analyzed.
RESULTS: Of the 763 children, 520 had eczema and 542 had atopy. Distributions of the genotype and allele frequencies of the HNMT 314C>T polymorphism were significantly associated with non-atopic eczema (P=0.004), and those of HNMT 939A>G were significantly associated with eczema in the atopy groups (P=0.048). Frequency distributions of HNMT -465T>C and -413C>T were not associated with eczema. Subjects who were AA homozygous or AG heterozygous for 939A>G showed significantly higher immunoglobulin E levels than subjects who were GG homozygous (P=0.009). In U937 cells, the variant genotype reporter construct had significantly higher mRNA stability (P<0.001) and HNMT enzyme activity (P<0.001) than the common genotype.
CONCLUSIONS: Polymorphisms in HNMT appear to confer susceptibility to AD in Korean children.

[What is histamine intolerance?] article in German: Was bedeutet Histaminintoleranz?
Lochner, S.
Medizinische Monatsschrift 35 Jahrgang 5/2012: 186-187
What is histamine intolerance? Which medicines can you take with this illness, which not?

Why all migraine patients should be treated with magnesium
Mauskop A, Varughese J
J Neural Transm. 2012 May; 119(5): 575-9
Magnesium, the second most abundant intracellular cation, is essential in many intracellular processes and appears to play an important role in migraine pathogenesis. Routine blood tests do not reflect true body magnesium stores since <2% is in the measurable, extracellular space, 67% is in the bone and 31% is located intracellularly. Lack of magnesium may promote cortical spreading depression, hyperaggregation of platelets, affect serotonin receptor function, and influence synthesis and release of a variety of neurotransmitters. Migraine sufferers may develop magnesium deficiency due to genetic inability to absorb magnesium, inherited renal magnesium wasting, excretion of excessive amounts of magnesium due to stress, low nutritional intake, and several other reasons. There is strong evidence that magnesium deficiency is much more prevalent in migraine sufferers than in healthy controls. Double-blind, placebo-controlled trials have produced mixed results, most likely because both magnesium deficient and non-deficient patients were included in these trials. This is akin to giving cyanocobalamine in a blinded fashion to a group of people with peripheral neuropathy without regard to their cyanocobalamine levels. Both oral and intravenous magnesium are widely available, extremely safe, very inexpensive and for patients who are magnesium deficient can be highly effective. Considering these features of magnesium, the fact that magnesium deficiency may be present in up to half of migraine patients, and that routine blood tests are not indicative of magnesium status, empiric treatment with at least oral magnesium is warranted in all migraine sufferers.

Effects of Amine Oxidases in Allergic and Histamine-Mediated Conditions
Mondovi B, Fogel WA, Federico R, Calinescu C, Mateescu MA, Rosa AC, Masini E
Recent Pat Inflamm Allergy Drug Discov. 2012
This review provides an update on histamine, on diamine oxidase (DAO) and on their implications in allergy and various conditions or affections, such as food histaminosis, ischemia and inflammatory bowel diseases (IBD). The review also

presents, in brief, patent coverage on therapies for allergy and IBD with the focus on histamine-related treatments.

Plasma diamine oxidase activity is a useful biomarker for evaluating gastrointestinal tract toxicities during chemotherapy with oral fluorouracil anti-cancer drugs in patients with gastric cancer
Namikawa T, Fukudome I, Kitagawa H, Okabayashi T, Kobayashi M, Hanazaki K.
Oncology. 2012; 82(3):147-52
OBJECTIVES: Diamine oxidase (DAO) is an enzyme that catalyzes oxidation and is highly active in the mature upper villus cells of the intestinal mucosa. This study sought to evaluate plasma DAO activities during adjuvant chemotherapy in patients with gastric cancer.
METHODS: We investigated 20 patients with gastric cancer who were treated with oral fluorouracil anti-cancer drugs as adjuvant chemotherapy. Plasma DAO activity was measured in all patients before chemotherapy and at 2, 4 and 6 weeks after the start of chemotherapy, and quality of life was evaluated simultaneously.
RESULTS: The median DAO activity after 4 weeks of chemotherapy was significantly decreased compared to the pre-chemotherapy levels (6.6 vs. 7.5 U/l; p = 0.038). The changes in the rate of DAO activity at 2 and 6 weeks following the start of chemotherapy in patients with gastrointestinal tract toxicity were significantly lower than in those without toxicity (p =0.021 and 0.047, respectively). The patient cohort showed a slightly positive correlation between DAO activity and global health status and a negative correlation between DAO activity and appetite loss.
CONCLUSIONS: Plasma DAO activities may be useful for monitoring and evaluating gastrointestinal tract toxicities induced by adjuvant chemotherapy with oral fluorouracil in patients with gastric cancer.

Histamine N-methyltransferase Thr105Ile polymorphism is associated with Parkinson's disease
Palada V, Terzić J, Mazzulli J, Bwala G, Hagenah J, Peterlin B, Hung AY, Klein C, Krainc D
Neurobiol Aging. 2012, 33(4): 836
Histamine is a central neurotransmitter degraded by histamine-N-methyltransferase (HNMT). Several abnormalities in the histaminergic system were found in patients with Parkinson's disease (PD), thus we tested the possible association of a Thr105Ile functional polymorphism in HNMT with PD. A total of 913 patients with PD and 958 controls were genotyped using a TaqMan RT-PCR Genotyping Assay (Foster City, California, USA). Lower frequency of HNMT Ile105 allele that is associated with decreased enzymatic activity was found in patients compared with controls ($\chi(2) = 11.65$; p = 0.0006). We performed meta-analysis to confirm the association of Thr105Ile functional polymorphism with PD. Our results indicate that lower HNMT activity plays a role in the pathogenesis of PD.

Structural brain changes in migraine
Palm-Meinders IH, Koppen H, Terwindt GM, Launer LJ, Konishi J, Moonen JM, Bakkers JT, Hofman PA, van Lew B, Middelkoop HA, van Buchem MA, Ferrari MD, Kruit MC
Journal of the American Medical Association (JAMA) 2012 Nov 14; 308(18): 1889-97
CONTEXT: A previous cross-sectional study showed an association of migraine with a higher prevalence of magnetic resonance imaging (MRI)-measured ischemic lesions in the brain.
OBJECTIVE: To determine whether women or men with migraine (with and without aura) have a higher incidence of brain lesions 9 years after initial MRI, whether migraine frequency was associated with progression of brain lesions, and whether progression of brain lesions was associated with cognitive decline.
DESIGN, SETTING, AND PARTICIPANTS: In a follow-up of the 2000 Cerebral Abnormalities in Migraine, an Epidemiological Risk Analysis cohort, a prospective population-based observational study of Dutch participants with migraine and an age- and sex-matched control group, 203 of the 295 baseline participants in the migraine group and 83 of 140 in the control group underwent MRI scan in 2009 to identify progression of MRI-measured brain lesions. Comparisons were adjusted for age, sex, hypertension, diabetes, and educational level. The participants in the migraine group were a mean 57 years (range, 43-72 years), and 71% were women. Those in the control group were a mean 55 years (range, 44-71 years), and 69% were women. MAIN OUTCOME MEASURES Progression of MRI-measured cerebral deep white matter hyperintensities, infratentorial hyperintensities, and posterior circulation territory infarctlike lesions. Change in cognition was also measured.
RESULTS: Of the 145 women in the migraine group, 112 (77%) vs 33 of 55 women (60%) in the control group had progression of deep white matter hyperintensities (adjusted odds ratio [OR], 2.1; 95%CI, 1.0-4.1; P = .04). There were no significant associations of migraine with progression of infratentorial hyperintensities: 21 participants (15%) in the migraine group and 1 of 57 participants (2%) in the control group showed progression (adjusted OR, 7.7; 95% CI, 1.0-59.5; P = .05) or new posterior circulation territory infarctlike lesions: 10 of 203 participants (5%) in the migraine group but none of 83 in the control group (P = .07). There was no association of number or frequency of migraine headaches with progression of lesions. There was no significant association of high vs nonhigh deep white matter hyperintensity load with change in cognitive scores (-3.7 in the migraine group vs 1.4 in the control group; 95% CI, -4.4 to 0.2; adjusted P = .07).

CONCLUSIONS: In a community-based cohort followed up after 9 years, women with migraine had a higher incidence of deep white matter hyperintensities but did not have significantly higher progression of other MRI-measured brain changes. There was no association of migraine with progression of any MRI-measured brain lesions in men.

Antimigraine (low-amine) diet may be helpful in children with cyclic vomiting syndrome
Paul SP, Barnard P, Soondrum K, Candy DC
J Pediatr Gastroenterol Nutr. 2012 May;54(5): 698-9
"Dietary modifications are frequently recommended for migraines. Given the overlapping features between migraines and cyclic vomiting syndrome (CVS), dietary treatments for CVS have aimed at eliminating trigger foods. Investigators from the UK describe a single center cohort of 21 children (2-16 years) were placed on a low-amine diet with instruction from a dietician (JPGN 2012; 54: 698-99). 16 (76%) of the children had a strong family history of migraines. The diet was implemented for a 'minimum of 6 to 8 weeks.' 13 had a complete resolution of vomiting and 18 (86%) had at least a partial response. Specific foods that were avoided included cheese, chocolate, citrus fruits, pork, peas, broad beans, shellfish, yeast extract, beef extract, gravies, caffeine, and alcohol."
Source: http://gutsandgrowth.wordpress.com/2012/07/02/diet-or-drugs-for-cyclic-vomiting-syndrome/#comment-424

Effect of omega-3 fatty acids on intensity of primary dysmenorrhea
Rahbar N, Asgharzadeh N, Ghorbani R.
Int J Gynaecol Obstet. 2012 Apr;117(1):45-7
OBJECTIVE: To examine whether dietary supplementation with omega-3 fatty acids relieved symptoms of primary dysmenorrhea.
METHODS: Women aged 18-22 years with primary dysmenorrhea were enrolled in a double-blind crossover study. Women assigned to group 1 (n=47) received 1 omega-3 capsule daily for 3 months, followed by placebo for 3 months. Women in group 2 (n=48) received placebo for 3 months, followed by omega-3 for 3 months. A washout period was performed in both groups. Participants used 400mg of ibuprofen as a rescue dose if severe menstrual pains were experienced.
RESULTS: A marked reduction in pain intensity was observed after 3 months of treatment with omega-3 fatty acids (P<0.05). Women who received omega-3 fatty acids required fewer rescue doses than women who received placebo (P<0.05). The mean numbers of ibuprofen tablets used after 3 months with omega-3 fatty acids were 4.3±2.1 (group 1) and 3.2±2.5 (group 2); the mean numbers of tablets used after 3 months of placebo were 5.3±2.2 (group 1) and 6.0±2.6 (group 2) (P=0.001 for both).
CONCLUSION: Supplementation with omega-3 fatty acids reduced the symptom intensity of primary dysmenorrhea. Supplementation efficacy was sufficient to decrease the ibuprofen rescue dose.

Leitlinie (Guidline) Vorgehen bei Verdacht auf Unverträglichkeit gegenüber oral aufgenommenem Histamin. Leitlinie der Deutschen Gesellschaft für Allergologie und klinische Immunologie (DGAKI), der Gesellschaft für Pädiatrische Allergologie und Umweltmedizin (GPA) und des Ärzteverbandes Deutscher Allergologen (ÄDA)
Reese I; Ballmer-Weber B; Beyer K; Erdmann S; Fuchs T; Kleine-Tebbe J; Klimek L; Lepp U; Henzgen M; Niggemann B; Saloga J; Schäfer C; Werfel T; Zuberbier T; Worm M.
Allergo J 2012; 21 (1): 22–28
Nahrungsmittelunverträglichkeiten sind deutlich seltener objektiv nachweisbar als subjektiv empfunden. Insbesondere zum wissenschaftlichen Kenntnisstand
nichtallergischer Überempfindlichkeitsreaktionen bestehen große Defizite. Ein Beispiel ist die Histaminunverträglichkeit, die aufgrund der starken Thematisierung in den Medien und im Internet von Betroffenen oftmals als Auslöser ihrer Gesundheitsbeschwerden vermutet wird. Die wissenschaftliche
Evidenz für die postulierten Zusammenhänge ist begrenzt, eine verlässliche Laborbestimmung zur definitiven Diagnose nicht vorhanden. Obwohl wissenschaftliche Untersuchungen zur Unverträglichkeit gegenüber exogen zugeführtem Histamin bisher ausschließlich bei Erwachsenen durchgeführt wurden, wird die Diagnose auch bei Kindern und Jugendlichen gestellt, mit oftmals einschneidenden Konsequenzen für den Speiseplan der Betroffenen. Die vorliegende Leitlinie der Arbeitsgruppe Nahrungs mittelallergie der Deutschen Gesellschaft für Allergologie und klinische Immunologie (DGAKI) in Zusammenarbeit mit dem Ärzteverband Deutscher Allergologen (ÄDA) und der Gesellschaft für Pädiatrische Allergologie und Umweltmedizin (GPA) fasst wichtige Aspekte zur Histaminunverträglichkeit und deren Konsequenzen für die Diagnostik und Therapie zusammen.

[Diagnostic and therapeutic procedure for two popular but quite distinct adverse reactions to food - fructose malabsorption and histamine intolerance]. [Article in German]
Reese I.
Ther Umsch. 2012 Apr; 69(4):231-7

Claiming to suffer from adverse food reactions is popular. In contrast to the classical food allergy, there are some pathomechanisms which are evidently dose-dependent. Thus the procedure in diagnosis and therapy must undoubtedly differ from the practice when food allergy is suspected or proven. Nevertheless many patients suffering from dose-dependent adversereactions to food are given strict elimination diets, which is neither necessary nor helpful and decreases their quality of life broadly. This holds especially true for fructose malabsorption and histamine intolerance. For the latter, the term adverse reaction to ingested histamine is preferred, because histamine intolerance implies that symptoms are caused entirely by an enzyme defect. Why this is not very likely to be the only reason is discussed in this article. Both adverse reactions require an individual approach especially with regard to nutrition therapy. Therefore the task of diagnosis should be to establish an individual profile of tolerated and not tolerated foods taking into account that tolerance can greatly vary by meal composition, frequency and individual triggering factors. In view of this, therapeutic recommendations should not be based on the absolute quantities of the eliciting substance to be eliminated but on a feasible transfer into daily life. Thereby food restriction can be minimized and a high quality of life will be maintained.

Biogenic amine production by the wine Lactobacillus brevis IOEB 9809 in systems that partially mimic the gastrointestinal tract stress

Russo P, Fernández de Palencia P, Romano A, Fernández M, Lucas P, Spano G, López P
BMC Microbiol. 2012 ; 12: 247

BACKGROUND: Ingestion of fermented foods containing high levels of biogenic amines (BA) can be deleterious to human health. Less obvious is the threat posed by BA producing organisms contained within the food which, in principle, could form BA after ingestion even if the food product itself does not initially contain high BA levels. In this work we have investigated the production of tyramine and putrescine by Lactobacillus brevis IOEB 9809, of wine origin, under simulated gastrointestinal tract (GIT) conditions.

RESULTS: An in vitro model that simulates the normal physiological conditions in the human digestive tract, as well as Caco-2 epithelial human cell lines, was used to challenge L. brevis IOEB 9809, which produced both tyramine and putrescine under all conditions tested. In the presence of BA precursors and under mild gastric stress, a correlation between enhancement of bacterial survival and a synchronous transcriptional activation of the tyramine and putrescine biosynthetic pathways was detected. High levels of both BA were observed after exposure of the bacterium to Caco-2 cells.

CONCLUSIONS: L. brevis IOEB 9809 can produce tyramine and putrescine under simulated human digestive tract conditions. The results indicate that BA production may be a mechanism that increases bacterial survival under gastric stress.

Unaltered histaminergic system in depression: A postmortem study

Shan L, Qi XR, Balesar R, Swaab DF, Bao AM.
J Affect Disord. 2012

BACKGROUND: Rodent experiments suggested that the neuronal histaminergic system may be involved in symptoms of depression.

METHODS: We determined, therefore, in postmortem tissue of 12 mood disorder patients (8 major depression disorder (MDD) and 4 bipolar disorder (BD)) and 12 well matched controls the expression of the rate-limiting enzyme for histamine production and histidine decarboxylase in the tuberomamillary nucleus (TMN) by quantitative in situ hybridization. In addition we used qPCR to determine the expression of the 4 histamine receptors and of the enzyme breaking down histamine, histamine N-methyltransferase (HMT), in the dorsolateral prefrontal cortex (DLPFC) and anterior cingulated cortex (ACC).

RESULTS: No changes were observed in the expression of these molecules, except for a significant lower HMT mRNA expression in the ACC of MDD subjects.

LIMITATIONS: Several inherent and potentially confounding factors of a postmortem study, such as medication and cause of death, did not seem to affect the conclusions. The group size was relatively small but well documented, both clinically and neuropathologically.

CONCLUSION: Except for a lower HMT mRNA expression in the ACC of MDD subjects, the neuronal histaminergic system did not show significant changes, either in the rate limiting enzyme involved in its production or in its receptors in 2 main projection sites, the ACC/DLPFC.

The effects of magnesium, L-carnitine, and concurrent magnesium-L-carnitine supplementation in migraine prophylaxis

Tarighat Esfanjani A, Mahdavi R, Ebrahimi Mameghani M, Talebi M, Nikniaz Z, Safaiyan A
Biol Trace Elem Res. 2012 Dec;150(1-3):42-8

Given the conflicting results about the positive effects of magnesium and L-carnitine and as there is no report concerning concurrent supplementation of magnesium and L-carnitine on migraine prophylaxis, the effects of magnesium, L-carnitine, and concurrent magnesium-L-carnitine supplementation on migraine indicators were assessed. In this clinical trial, 133 migrainous patients were randomly assigned into three intervention groups: magnesium oxide (500 mg/day), L-carnitine (500 mg/day), and Mg-L-carnitine (500 mg/day magnesium and 500 mg/day L-carnitine), and a control group. After 12 weeks of supplementation, the checklist of migraine indicators including migraine attacks/month, migraine days/month, and headache severity was completed, and serum concentrations of magnesium and L-carnitine were measured by atomic absorption spectrophotometry and enzymatic UV test, respectively. The results showed a significant reduction in all migraine indicators in all studied groups ($p < 0.05$). The ANOVA results showed a significant reduction in migraine frequency across various supplemented and control groups ($p = 0.008$). By separating the effects of magnesium supplementation from other confounding factors such as routine treatments using the repeated measures and nested model, it was clarified that magnesium supplementation had a significant effect on all migraine indicators. Oral supplementation with magnesium oxide and L-carnitine and concurrent supplementation of Mg-L-carnitine besides routine treatments could be effective in migraine prophylaxis; however, larger trials are needed to confirm these preliminary findings.

Definitions, criteria and global classification of mast cell disorders with special reference to mast cell activation syndromes: a consensus proposal

Valent P, Akin C, Arock M, Brockow K, Butterfield JH, Carter MC, Castells M, Escribano L, Hartmann K, Lieberman P, Nedoszytko B, Orfao A, Schwartz LB, Sotlar K, Sperr WR, Triggiani M, Valenta R, Horny HP, Metcalfe DD

Int Arch Allergy Immunol. 2012;157(3):215-25

Activation of tissue mast cells (MCs) and their abnormal growth and accumulation in various organs are typically found in primary MC disorders also referred to as mastocytosis. However, increasing numbers of patients are now being informed that their clinical findings are due to MC activation (MCA) that is neither associated with mastocytosis nor with a defined allergic or inflammatory reaction. In other patients with MCA, MCs appear to be clonal cells, but criteria for diagnosing mastocytosis are not met. A working conference was organized in 2010 with the aim to define criteria for diagnosing MCA and related disorders, and to propose a global unifying classification of all MC disorders and pathologic MC reactions. This classification includes three types of 'MCA syndromes' (MCASs), namely primary MCAS, secondary MCAS and idiopathic MCAS. MCA is now defined by robust and generally applicable criteria, including (1) typical clinical symptoms, (2) a substantial transient increase in serum total tryptase level or an increase in other MC-derived mediators, such as histamine or prostaglandin D(2), or their urinary metabolites, and (3) a response of clinical symptoms to agents that attenuate the production or activities of MC mediators. These criteria should assist in the identification and diagnosis of patients with MCAS, and in avoiding misdiagnoses or overinterpretation of clinical symptoms in daily practice. Moreover, the MCAS concept should stimulate research in order to identify and exploit new molecular mechanisms and therapeutic targets.

[Histamine Intolerance Syndrome (HIS): Plethora of Physiological, Pathophysiological and Toxic Mechanisms and their Differentiation] [Article in German]

Weidenhiller M, Layritz C, Hagel AF, Kuefner M, Zopf Y, Raithel M

Z Gastroenterol. 2012; 50(12): 1302-9

BACKGROUND: Non-immunological types of foodstuffs intolerance are reported by about 15-20% people of the population. The intolerance of histamine and to some extent of other biogenic amines (such as cadaverine, putrescine, tyramine etc.) plays an important role in the differential diagnosis of the foodstuff intolerances and has to be strictly separated from immunologically mediated foodstuffs reactions (foodstuffs allergies, 2-5% of the population).
METHODS: Clinical data from the Erlangen interdisciplinary data register of allergic and chronic inflammatory gastro-intestinal diseases were analysed respecting the existence of a histamine intolerance, then classified and summarised; in addition a selective literature research was undertaken in May 2011.
RESULTS: In non-immunological cases of foodstuffs intolerance, the patient´s intolerance of histamine plays quite a significant role, clinically it has been exactly proven only in a small subgroup of patients by standardised blinded provocation reactions. The histamine intolerance syndrome (HIS) often presents in a non-specific manner and has to be separated from other pseudo-allergic reactions, idiopathic intolerance reactions, organic differential diagnosis (for example, chronic infections, allergies, mastocytosis etc.) as well as medicamentous adverse effects and psychosomatic reactions.
CONCLUSION: The clinical picture of histamine intolerance should be definitely assured, after the exclusion of other differential diagnosis, by standardised histamine provocation. The avoidance of histamine and biogenic amines, the use of antihistaminics and the instauration of a proportionate nutrient matter are the most important therapeutic options next to a detailed education of the patient.

A Case of Histamine Fish Poisoning in a Young Atopic Woman

Wilson BJ, Musto RJ, Ghali WA

J Gen Intern Med. 2012 Jan 31

Histamine fish poisoning, also known as scombroid poisoning, is a histamine toxicity syndrome that results from eating specific types of spoiled fish. Although typically a benign syndrome, characterized by self-limited flushing, headache, and gastrointestinal symptoms, we describe a case unique in its severity and as a precipitant of an asthma exacerbation. A 25-year-old woman presented to the emergency department (ED) with one hour of tongue and face swelling, an erythematous pruritic rash, and dyspnea with wheezing after consuming a tuna sandwich. She developed abdominal pain, diarrhea and hypotension in the ED requiring admission to the hospital. A diagnosis of histamine fish poisoning was made and the patient was treated supportively and discharged within 24 hours, but was readmitted within 3 hours due to an asthma exacerbation. Her course was complicated by recurrent admissions for asthma exacerbations.

2011

Treatment of Atopic Dermatitis with a Low-histamine Diet
Chung BY, Cho SI, Ahn IS, Lee HB, Kim HO, Park CW, Lee CH.
Ann Dermatol. 2011 Sep; 23 Suppl 1: S91-5

Atopic dermatitis (AD) has numerous trigger factors. The question of whether foods can aggravate AD remains open to debate. Although a number of published papers have detailed the relationship between food allergies and AD, little research has examined the question of how food intolerance affects AD. For the purposes of this study, a six-year-old Korean boy with AD was admitted to the hospital for evaluation of the possibility of food, particularly pork, as a triggering factor in his skin disease. He had a history of worsening of symptoms when eating pork. Total serum IgE concentration was 157 IU/ml. House dust was class 2.2 (1.5 IU/ml) in MAST. All other MAST items were negative. In an oral food challenge test, he showed a positive result after eating 200 g of pork, but did not show a positive result after eating 60 g of pork. After discharge, we attempted to keep him on a balanced diet that included various types of food and prohibited him from eating food that contains a high level of histamine. After keeping the patient on a balanced and low-histamine dietary regimen, his AD symptoms showed improvement and have not worsened for more than seven months. A low-histamine, balanced diet could be helpful for AD patients having symptoms that resemble histamine intolerance in which their AD symptoms worsened after intake of histamine-rich foods, but in which food allergy tests are negative.

Scientific Opinion on risk based control of biogenic amine formation in fermented foods
EFSA Panel on Biological Hazards (BIOHAZ)
EFSA Journal 2011;9(10): 2393, [93 pp.]

A qualitative risk assessment of biogenic amines (BA) in fermented foods was conducted, using data from the scientific literature, as well as from European Union-related surveys, reports and consumption data. Histamine and tyramine are considered as the most toxic and food safety relevant, and fermented foods are of particular BA concern due to associated intensive microbial activity and potential for BA formation. Based on mean content in foods and consumer exposure data, fermented food categories were ranked in respect to histamine and tyramine, but presently available information was insufficient to conduct quantitative risk assessment of BA, individually and in combination(s). Regarding BA risk mitigation options, particularly relevant are hygienic measures to minimize the occurrence of BA-producing microorganisms in raw material, additional microbial controls and use of BAnonproducing starter cultures. Based on limited published information, no adverse health effects were observed after exposure to following BA levels in food (per person per meal): a) 50 mg histamine for healthy individuals, but below detectable limits for those with histamine intolerance; b) 600 mg tyramine for healthy individuals not taking monoamino oxidase inhibitor (MAOI) drugs, but 50 mg for those taking third generation MAOI drugs or 6 mg for those taking classical MAOI drugs; and c) for putrescine and cadaverine, the information was insufficient in that respect. Presently, only high-performance liquid chromatography (HPLC)-based methods enable simultaneous and high sensitivity quantification of all BA in foods, hence are best suited for monitoring and control purposes. Monitoring of BA concentrations in fermented foods during the production process and along the food chain would be beneficial for controls and further knowledge. Further research on BA in fermented foods is needed; particularly on toxicity and associated concentrations, production process-based control measures, further process hygiene and/or food safety criteria development, and validation of analysis methods.

Role of tyramine synthesis by food-borne Enterococcus durans in adaptation to the gastrointestinal tract environment
Fernández de Palencia P, Fernández M, Mohedano ML, Ladero V, Quevedo C, Alvarez MA, López P.
Appl Environ Microbiol. 2011 Jan; 77(2): 699-702

Biogenic amines in food constitute a human health risk. Here we report that tyramine-producing Enterococcus durans strain IPLA655 (from cheese) was able to produce tyramine under conditions simulating transit through the gastrointestinal tract. Activation of the tyramine biosynthetic pathway contributed to binding and immunomodulation of enterocytes.

[Diamine oxidase as blood biomarker in rats and humans to GI tract toxicity of fluorouracil anti-cancer drugs]. [Article in Japanese]
Goto T, Matsubara T, Yoshizawa Y, Sasaya S, Nemoto H, Sanada Y, Moriyama K, Kouchi Y.

Gan To Kagaku Ryoho. 2011; 38(5): 765-9
Diarrhea is a side effect of a 5-fluorouracil (5-FU) anti-cancer drug-induced intestinal mucosal disorder, which sometimes becomes more severe. Blood diamine oxidase (DAO; EC1. 4. 3. 6) activity is reported to be significantly correlated with activity in the small intestinal mucosal tissue, and to be a reliable indicator of small intestinal mucosal integrity and maturity. Here, we investigated whether blood DAO activity can be a biomarker for the gastrointestinal (GI) mucosal disorder caused by 5-FU anti-cancer drugs, both in rats and humans. From results of the rat study, the degree of jejunal mucosal disorder caused by the 5-FU anti-cancer drug was well correlated with a decrease in blood DAO activity. Clinically, 12 out of 28 patients (43%) administered 5-FU anti-cancer drug suffered from diarrhea. The plasma DAO activity within one week of the onset of diarrhea significantly decreased compared with that before the administration. Furthermore, before drug administration, plasma DAO activity in patients suffering from diarrhea was higher than those in patients without diarrhea. Although DAO activity differs by the individual, it is a useful biomarker for estimating the degree of intestinal mucosal disorder, and possibly for estimating manifestations of diarrhea induced by 5-FU anti-cancer drug administration.

Mast cell activation syndrome: a newly recognized disorder with systemic clinical manifestations

Hamilton MJ, Hornick JL, Akin C, Castells MC, Greenberger NJ
J Allergy Clin Immunol. 2011; 128(1): 147-152

BACKGROUND: Diagnostic criteria for mast cell (MC) activation syndrome have been recently proposed, but clinical studies to validate these criteria are lacking.
OBJECTIVE: We sought to determine the clinical manifestations of this newly recognized syndrome in a cohort of patients.
METHODS: We prospectively evaluated 18 patients seen at our institution with MC activation syndrome from 2006 to 2009. Patients enrolled had at least 4 of the signs and symptoms of abdominal pain, diarrhea, flushing, dermatographism, memory and concentration difficulties, or headache. Response to treatment with anti-MC mediator medications was assessed based on established criteria. Laboratory tests indicating MC mediator release and histopathology and immunohistochemical studies on gastrointestinal biopsy samples were performed.
RESULTS: Ninety-four percent of the patients had abdominal pain, 89% had dermatographism, 89% had flushing, and 72% had the constellation of all 3 symptoms. Patients additionally had headache, diarrhea, and memory and concentration difficulties. All patients had at least 1 positive laboratory test result for an increased MC mediator level. On the basis of the response to treatment criteria, 67% of the patients in the cohort had either a complete or major regression in symptoms while taking medications targeting MC mediators. There was no significant difference in the numbers of intestinal mucosal MCs between our patients and healthy control subjects.
CONCLUSION: MC activation syndrome might be the underlying cause of unexplained symptoms when several organ systems are involved, such as the gastrointestinal tract and the skin. It is especially important to be able to recognize the constellation of clinical features because response to anti-MC mediator medications is often excellent.

Evaluation of Helicobacter pylori infection in patients with common migraine headache

Hosseinzadeh M, Khosravi A, Saki K, Ranjbar R
Arch Med Sci. 2011; 7(5): 844-9

INTRODUCTION: Migraine can cause headache in different communities so that 12-15% are suffering worldwide. Recently the relationship between infectious diseases such as Helicobacter pylori infection and migraine headache has been the focus of many studies. The current study was designed to evaluate IgG and IgM antibodies to H. pylori in patients suffering from migraine headaches.
MATERIAL AND METHODS: Patients who had diagnostic criteria for migraine were chosen as cases compared to some healthy individuals as the control group amongst which immunoglobulin G (IgG), immunoglobulin M (IgM), age, job, gastro-intestinal (GI) disorders, history of migraine, special meals, medications, sleeping disorders, stress, environmental factors etc were analysed.
RESULTS: The prevalence of disease was 38.6%. Household women had the highest prevalence (40%). Among them menstruation was related to high prevalence of migraine. 75.6% of patients had gastrointestinal disorders of which the gastric reflux was the most important sign (47.1%). The mean optical density (OD) value of IgG and IgM antibody to H. pylori was 60.08 ±7.7 and 32.1 ±8.7 for the case group, 21.82 ±6.2 and 17.6 ±9.4 for the control group, respectively.
CONCLUSIONS: There was a significant difference in mean OD value of both antibodies to H. pylori amongst the case and control groups. As a result, active H. pylori infection is strongly related to the outbreak and severity of migraine headaches, and H. pylori treatment reduces migraine headaches significantly. Hopefully, the definite treatment and eradication of this infection can cure or reduce the severity and course of migraine headaches significantly if not totally.

Clinial study. Histamine 50-skin-prick test: a tool to diagnose histamine intolerance

L. Kofler, H. Ulmer, H. Kofler
ISRN Allergy, volume 2011, article ID 353045, 5 pages (open access article)

BACKGROUND. Histamine intolerance results from an imbalance between histamine intake and degradation. In healthy persons, dietary histamine can be sufficiently metabolized by amine oxidases, whereas persons with low amine oxidase activity are at risk of histamine toxicity. Diamine oxidase (DAO) is the key enzyme in degradation. Histamine elicits a wide range of effects. Histamine intolerance displays symptoms, such as rhinitis, headache, gastrointestinal symptoms, palpitations, urticaria and pruritus. OBJECTIVE. Diagnosis of histamine intolerance until now is based on case history; neither a validated questionnaire nor a routine test is available. It was the aim of this trial to evaluate the usefullness of a prick-test for the diagnosis of histamine intolerance. METHODS. Prick-testing with 1% histamine solution and wheal size-measurement to assess the relation between the wheal in prick-test, read after 20 to 50 minutes, as sign of slowed histamine degradation as well as history and symptoms of histamine intolerance. RESULST. Besides a pretest with 17 patients with HIT we investigated 156 persons (81 with HIT, 75 controls): 64 out of 81 with histamine intolerance(HIT), but only 14 out of 75 persons from the control-group presented with a histamine wheal ≥3mmafter 50minutes (P < .0001). CONCLUSIONS AND CLINICAL RELEVANCE. Histamine-50 skin-prickt-test offers a simple tool with relevance.

EU survey and results about mastocytosis, survey 2010
König A
2011
http://www.mastozytose.com/European%20results%20survey%202010.pdf

Final report of the BIAMFOOD project: Controlling Biogenic Amines in Traditional Food Fermentations in Regional Europe (EU Project 211441)
Lolkema J. (project coordinator, Groningen University)
2011

Association of single nucleotide polymorphisms in the diamine oxidase gene with diamine oxidase serum activities
Maintz L, Yu CF, Rodríguez E, Baurecht H, Bieber T, Illig T, Weidinger S, Novak N
Allergy. 2011 Apr 13
BACKGROUND: Histamine intolerance (HIT) is associated with an excess of histamine because of an impaired function of the histamine-degrading enzyme diamine oxidase (DAO). The genetic background of HIT is unknown yet.
METHODS: Case-control association study of all haplotype tagging and four previously reported DAO SNPs and one HNMT Single nucleotide polymorphism with symptoms of HIT and DAO serum activity in 484 German individuals including 285 patients with clinical symptoms of HIT and 199 controls.
RESULTS: Diamine oxidase serum activity was significantly associated with seven SNPs within the DAO gene. The minor allele at rs2052129, rs2268999, rs10156191 and rs1049742 increased the risk for a reduced DAO activity whereas showing a moderate protective effect at rs2071514, rs1049748 and rs2071517 in the genotypic (P $=$ 2.1 $\times$ $10(-8)$, 7.6 $\times$ $10(-10)$, 8.3 $\times$ $10(-10)$, 0.009, 0.005, 0.00001, 0.006, respectively) and allelic genetic model (P $=$ 2.5 $\times$ $10(-11)$, 5.4 $\times$ $10(-13)$, 8.9 $\times$ $10(-13)$, 0.00002, 0.006, 0.0003, 0.005, respectively). Reporter gene assays at rs2052129 revealed a lower promoter activity (P $=$ 0.016) of the minor allele. DAO mRNA expression in peripheral blood mononuclear cells of homozygous carriers of the minor allele at rs2052129, rs2268999, rs10156191 was lower (P $=$ 0.002) than homozygous carriers of the major allele. Diamine oxidase variants were not associated with the HIT phenotype per se, only with DAO activity alone and the subgroup of HIT patients displaying a reduced DAO activity.
CONCLUSIONS: DAO gene variants strongly influence DAO expression and activity but alone are not sufficient to fully effectuate the potentially associated disease state of HIT, suggesting an interplay of genetic and environmental factors.

No association between histamine N-methyltransferase functional polymorphism Thr105Ile and Alzheimer's disease
Marasović-Šušnjara I, Palada V, Marinović-Terzić I, Mimica N, Marin J, Muck-Seler D, Mustapić M, Presečki P, Pivac N, Folnegović-Šmalc V, Marinović-Ćurin J, Terzić J.
Neurosci Lett. 2011, 489(2): 119-21
Several abnormalities, including lower histamine levels in brain, elevated serum histamine and degeneration of histaminergic neurons in tuberomammillary nucleus, were described in the histaminergic system of patients with Alzheimer's disease (AD). Histamine is a central neurotransmitter with several functions in brain including regulation of memory, cognition, locomotion, and is degraded in part by histamine N-methyltransferase (HNMT). A common Thr105Ile polymorphism within HNMT gene results in decreased enzyme activity. The Thr105Ile polymorphism was associated with Parkinson's disease, essential tremor, attention-deficit hyperactivity disorder (ADHD), asthma and alcoholism, thus we tested possible association of HNMT functional polymorphism with AD. We have tested 256 AD cases and 1190 healthy controls of Croatian origin. Thr105Ile polymorphism was determined by TaqMan RT-PCR Genotyping Assay and EcoRV digestion. Prevalence

of functional HNMT polymorphism among all tested groups was similar and frequency of less active Ile105 variant was 11.5% among AD patients and 13.4% for healthy controls (p=0.26, X(2)=1.25). Our results indicate lack of the association of HNMT Thr105Ile functional polymorphism with Alzheimer's disease.

[Nutrition therapy for adverse reactions to histamine in food and beverages] Ernährungstherapie bei Unverträglichkeit gegenüber oral aufgenommenem Histamin
Reese, I.
Allergologie, Jahrgang 34, Nr. 3/2011, S. 152–158
Adverse reactions to food are suspected in one third of the German population, but only 10% of these assumed hypersensitivity reactions can be clinically confirmed. While diagnosis of food allergies is fairly easy due to objective laboratory parameters, non-allergic hypersensitivity reactions are difficult to diagnose because these objective markers are lacking so far. Adverse reactions to histamine are often suspected to be the cause of a wide range of symptoms, especially when no allergic pathomechanism can be identified. In order to confirm such a suspicion, it is inevitable to validate a reproducible association between consumption of food and beverages rich in histamine and symptoms, to identify causative agents and to exclude other disorders. Thereafter, avoidance should be performed on the basis of individual requirements. General advices with a lot of restraints are often unnecessarily strict. Nutrition therapy aims at a reduction of symptoms to a minimum while maintaining a high quality of life.

Primary headache syndromes in systemic mastocytosis
Smith JH, Butterfield JH, Cutrer FM
Cephalalgia. 2011; 31(15): 1522-31
AIM: To investigate the relationship between clinical mast cell activity and primary headache syndromes.
METHODS: We surveyed individuals with systemic mastocytosis, an uncommon disorder associated with increased mast cell activity. Diagnoses of primary headache syndromes in addition to the relationship of headache and symptoms of mastocytosis were ascertained.
RESULTS: A response rate of 64/148 (43.2%) was achieved. Headache diagnoses in our respondents (n = 64) were largely migraine (37.5%) and tension-type headaches (17.2%). Typical aura with and without migraine headache was highly represented in our patient population (n = 25, 39%). Three individuals met criteria for primary cough headache (4.7%). Symptoms reflective of mast cell activity were significantly greater in individuals reporting headaches. Patients experiencing headache concurrently with mastocytosis flairs were more likely to be male (p = 0.002), have histaminergic symptoms, such as itching (p = 0.02) and runny nose (p = 0.03), and have unilateral cranial autonomic features (p = 0.04). However, using standardized International Headache Society criteria, we did not identify individuals with cluster headache or other trigeminal autonomic cephalalgias in this population.
CONCLUSIONS: Our observational survey-based data supports a clinical relationship between mast cell activity and primary headache syndromes. Generalizability of our results is limited by the low response rate and possible tertiary referral bias.

Neurologic symptoms and diagnosis in adults with mast cell disease
Smith JH, Butterfield JH, Pardanani A, DeLuca GC, Cutrer FM
Clin Neurol Neurosurg. 2011; 113(7): 570-4
OBJECTIVE: To identify complications of mastocytosis that impact the nervous system across a large cohort.
PATIENTS AND METHODS: In this retrospective series, we reviewed the electronic medical records of adult patients with a diagnosis of mastocytosis who were referred to a Neurologist at Mayo Clinic in Rochester, MN from January 1, 1999 to December 31, 2008.
RESULTS: Thirty patients were identified who presented to a Neurologist with symptoms potentially related to the mast cell disease. Twelve of these patients presented with complex spells involving syncope, which frequently preceded a formal diagnosis of mastocytosis. Nine individuals presented with acute back pain which was ultimately deemed symptomatic of vertebral compression fractures. One individual experienced spinal cord compression from a vertebral mast cell infiltrate. Headaches were reported in 78/223 (35%) total patients with mastocytosis. Although details of headaches were insufficiently ascertained to diagnose most, the five individuals in our referral cohort met International Headache Society (IHS) criteria for migraine. Finally, three individuals (1.3%) were identified with multiple sclerosis occurring at variable times after the mast cell diagnosis.
CONCLUSION: Symptoms related to mastocytosis may be encountered by neurologists and mimic many common, often idiopathic syndromes including, syncopal spells, back pain, and headache. In our cohort, multiple sclerosis may be over-represented. Mastocytosis should be considered in patients with these presentations, especially when also accompanied by flushing, abdominal cramping or diarrhea.

Quantitative Determination of Acetaldehyde in Foods Using Automated Digestion with Simulated Gastric Fluid Followed by Headspace Gas Chromatography
Uebelacker M, Lachenmeier DW
J Autom Methods Manag Chem. 2011; 2011: 907317
Acetaldehyde (ethanal) is a genotoxic carcinogen, which may occur naturally or as an added flavour in foods. We have developed an efficient method to analyze the compound in a wide variety of food matrices. The analysis is conducted using headspace (HS) gas chromatography (GC) with flame ionization detector. Using a robot autosampler, the samples are digested in full automation with simulated gastric fluid (1h at 37°C) under shaking, which frees acetaldehyde loosely bound to matrix compounds. Afterwards, an aliquot of the HS is injected into the GC system. Standard addition was applied for quantification to compensate for matrix effects. The precision of the method was sufficient (<3% coefficient of variation). The limit of detection was 0.01mg/L and the limit of quantification was 0.04mg/L. 140 authentic samples were analyzed. The acetaldehyde content in apples was 0.97 ± 0.80mg/kg, orange juice contained 3.86 ± 2.88mg/kg. The highest concentration was determined in a yoghurt (17mg/kg). A first-exposure estimation resulted in a daily acetaldehyde intake of less than 0.1mg/kg bodyweight from food, which is considerably lower than the exposures from alcohol consumption or tobacco smoking.

The histamine H_4 receptor: targeting inflammatory disorders
Walter M, Kottke T, Stark H
Eur J Pharmacol. 2011;668(1-2): 1-5
The discovery of the histamine H(4) receptor has added a new chapter to the century of extensive biogenic amine research. The human histamine H(4) receptor is mainly expressed in cells of the human immune system (e.g. mast cells, eosinophils, monocytes, dendritic cells, T cells) and mediates several effects on chemotaxis with numerous cell types. The distinct expression pattern and the immunomodulatory role highlight its physiological relevance in inflammatory and immunological processes. Inflammatory conditions, e.g. allergy, asthma and autoimmune diseases, were for a long time thought to be mainly mediated by activation of the histamine H(1) receptor subtype. However, in the treatment of diseases as chronic pruritus, asthma and allergic rhinitis the use of histamine H(1) receptor antagonists is unsatisfying. Selective H(4) receptor ligands and/or synergism of histamine H(1) and H(4) receptor modulation may be more effective in such pathophysiological conditions. Promising preclinical studies underline its role as an attractive target in the treatment of inflammatory and autoimmune disorders. Meanwhile, first histamine H(4) receptor antagonist has reached clinical phases for the treatment of respiratory diseases.

2010

Mast cell activation syndrome: Proposed diagnostic criteria
Akin C, Valent P, Metcalfe DD
J Allergy Clin Immunol. 2010; 126(6):1099-104
The term mast cell activation syndrome (MCAS) is finding increasing use as a diagnosis for subjects who present with signs and symptoms involving the dermis, gastrointestinal track, and cardiovascular system frequently accompanied by neurologic complaints. Such patients often have undergone multiple extensive medical evaluations by different physicians in varied disciplines without a definitive medical diagnosis until the diagnosis of MCAS is applied. However, MCAS as a distinct clinical entity has not been generally accepted, nor do there exist definitive criteria for diagnosis. Based on current understanding of this disease "syndrome" and on what we do know about mast cell activation and resulting pathology, we will explore and propose criteria for its diagnosis. The proposed criteria will be discussed in the context of other disorders involving mast cells or with similar presentations and as a basis for further scientific study and validation.

Diet restriction in migraine, based on IgG against foods: a clinical double-blind, randomised, cross-over trial
Alpay K, Ertas M, Orhan EK, Ustay DK, Lieners C, Baykan B
Cephalalgia. 2010; 30(7): 829-37
INTRODUCTION: It is well-known that specific foods trigger migraine attacks in some patients. We aimed to investigate the effect of diet restriction, based on IgG antibodies against food antigens on the course of migraine attacks in this randomised, double blind, cross-over, headache-diary based trial on 30 patients diagnosed with migraine without aura.
METHODS: Following a 6-week baseline, IgG antibodies against 266 food antigens were detected by ELISA. Then, the patients were randomised to a 6-week diet either excluding or including specific foods with raised IgG antibodies, individually. Following a 2-week diet-free interval after the first diet period, the same patients were given the opposite 6-week diet (provocation diet following elimination diet or vice versa). Patients and their physicians were blinded to IgG test results and the type of diet (provocation or elimination). Primary parameters were number of headache days and migraine attack count. Of 30 patients, 28 were female and 2 were male, aged 19-52 years (mean, 35 +/- 10 years).

RESULTS: The average count of reactions with abnormally high titre was 24 +/- 11 against 266 foods. Compared to baseline, there was a statistically significant reduction in the number of headache days (from 10.5 +/- 4.4 to 7.5 +/- 3.7; P < 0.001) and number of migraine attacks (from 9.0 +/- 4.4 to 6.2 +/- 3.8; P < 0.001) in the elimination diet period.
CONCLUSION: This is the first randomised, cross-over study in migraineurs, showing that diet restriction based on IgG antibodies is an effective strategy in reducing the frequency of migraine attacks.

Histamine-N-methyl transferase polymorphism and risk for multiple sclerosis

García-Martín E, Martínez C, Benito-León J, Calleja P, Díaz-Sánchez M, Pisa D, Alonso-Navarro H, Ayuso-Peralta L, Torrecilla D, Agúndez JA, Jiménez-Jiménez FJ.
Eur J Neurol. 2010, 17(2): 335-8

BACKGROUND: Histamine N-methyltransferase (HNMT) is the main metabolizing enzyme of histamine (a mediator of inflammation implicated in the pathogenesis of multiple sclerosis-MS) in the CNS. We have investigated the possible association between a single nucleotide polymorphism of the HNMT (chromosome 2q22.1), that causes the amino acid substitution Thr105Ile (decreasing enzyme activity) and the risk for MS.
METHODS: We studied the frequency of the HNMT genotypes and allelic variants in 228 MS patients and 295 healthy controls using a PCR-RLFP method.
RESULTS: The frequencies of the HNMT genotypes and allelic variants did not differ significantly between MS patients and controls, and were unrelated with the age of onset of MS, gender, and course of MS.
CONCLUSION: The HNMT polymorphism is not related with the risk for MS.

Vitamin B6 is required for full motility and virulence in Helicobacter pylori

Grubman A, Phillips A, Thibonnier M, Kaparakis-Liaskos M, Johnson C, Thiberge JM, Radcliff FJ, Ecobichon C, Labigne A, de Reuse H, Mendz GL, Ferrero RL
MBio. 2010 Aug 17; 1(3)

Despite recent advances in our understanding of how Helicobacter pylori causes disease, the factors that allow this pathogen to persist in the stomach have not yet been fully characterized. To identify new virulence factors in H. pylori, we generated low-infectivity variants of a mouse-colonizing H. pylori strain using the classical technique of in vitro attenuation. The resulting variants and their highly infectious progenitor bacteria were then analyzed by global gene expression profiling. The gene expression levels of five open reading frames (ORFs) were significantly reduced in low-infectivity variants, with the most significant changes observed for ORFs HP1583 and HP1582. These ORFs were annotated as encoding homologs of the Escherichia coli vitamin B(6) biosynthesis enzymes PdxA and PdxJ. Functional complementation studies with E. coli confirmed H. pylori PdxA and PdxJ to be bona fide homologs of vitamin B(6) biosynthesis enzymes. Importantly, H. pylori PdxA was required for optimal growth in vitro and was shown to be essential for chronic colonization in mice. In addition to having a well-known metabolic role, vitamin B(6) is necessary for the synthesis of glycosylated flagella and for flagellum-based motility in H. pylori. Thus, for the first time, we identify vitamin B(6) biosynthesis enzymes as novel virulence factors in bacteria. Interestingly, pdxA and pdxJ orthologs are present in a number of human pathogens, but not in mammalian cells. We therefore propose that PdxA/J enzymes may represent ideal candidates for therapeutic targets against bacterial pathogens.

Scombroid poisoning: a review

Hungerford JM
Source: Toxicon 56 (2010) 231-243

Scombroid poisoning, also called histamine fish poisoning, is an allergy-like form of food poisoning that continues to be a major problem in seafood safety. The exact role of histamine in scombroid poisoning is not straightforward. Deviations from the expected dose-response have led to the advancement of various possible mechanisms of toxicity, none of them proven. Histamine action levels are used in regulation until more is known about the mechanism of scombroid poisoning. Scombroid poisoning and histamine are correlated but complicated. Victims of scombroid poisoning respond well to antihistamines, and chemical analyses of fish implicated in scombroid poisoning generally reveal elevated levels of histamine. Scombroid poisoning is unique among the seafood toxins since it results from product mishandling rather than contamination from other trophic levels. Inadequate cooling following harvest promotes bacterial histamine production, and can result in outbreaks of scombroid poisoning. Fish with high levels of free histidine, the enzyme substrate converted to histamine by bacterial histidine decarboxylase, are those most often implicated in scombroid poisoning. Laboratory methods and screening methods for detecting histamine are available in abundance, but need to be compared and validated to harmonize testing. Successful field testing, including dockside or on-board testing needed to augment HACCP efforts will have to integrate rapid and simplified detection methods with simplified and rapid sampling and extraction. Otherwise, time-consuming sample preparation reduces the impact of gains in detection speed on the overall analysis time.

Estradiol and progesterone regulate the migration of mast cells from the periphery to the uterus and induce their maturation and degranulation

Jensen F, Woudwyk M, Teles A, Woidacki K, Taran F, Costa S, Malfertheiner SF, Zenclussen AC.

Source: PLoS One. 2010 Dec 22;5(12):e14409

BACKGROUND: Mast cells (MCs) have long been suspected as important players for implantation based on the fact that their degranulation causes the release of pivotal factors, e.g., histamine, MMPs, tryptase and VEGF, which are known to be involved in the attachment and posterior invasion of the embryo into the uterus. Moreover, MC degranulation correlates with angiogenesis during pregnancy. The number of MCs in the uterus has been shown to fluctuate during menstrual cycle in human and estrus cycle in rat and mouse indicating a hormonal influence on their recruitment from the periphery to the uterus. However, the mechanisms behind MC migration to the uterus are still unknown.

METHODOLOGY/PRINCIPAL FINDINGS: We first utilized migration assays to show that MCs are able to migrate to the uterus and to the fetal-maternal interface upon up-regulation of the expression of chemokine receptors by hormonal changes. By using a model of ovariectomized animals, we provide clear evidences that also in vivo, estradiol and progesterone attract MC to the uterus and further provoke their maturation and degranulation.

CONCLUSION/SIGNIFICANCE: We propose that estradiol and progesterone modulate the migration of MCs from the periphery to the uterus and their degranulation, which may prepare the uterus for implantation.

Fruits and Fruit Flavor: Classification and Biological Characterization

Jiang YM, Song J.

Chapter 1 in: Handbook of Fruit and Vegetable Flavors, Edited by Y. H. Hui, John Wiley & Sons 2010

Histamine N-methyltransferase Thr105Ile is not associated with Parkinson's disease or essential tremor

Keeling BH, Vilariño-Güell C, Soto-Ortolaza AI, Ross OA, Uitti RJ, Rajput A, Wszolek ZK, Farrer MJ

Parkinsonism Relat Disord. 2010, 16(2): 112-4

A functional variant in the Histamine N-Methyltransferase gene (HNMT - rs11558538) resulting in a threonine to isoleucine substitution (Thr105Ile) has been shown to impair histamine degradation. Two recent studies reported that the threonine allele of this polymorphism might be a risk factor for Parkinson disease (PD) and essential tremor (ET) development. Although PD and ET are considered different entities, they share some clinical and pathological features, suggesting a possible joint etiology. In this study we assess the role of the Thr105Ile variant in PD and ET development, genotyping the variant in a North American Caucasian PD and ET case-control series. Statistical analysis did not identify any significant association between this variant and PD or ET; therefore, our findings do not support the HNMT Thr105Ile variant as a factor in disease development or a genetic link between the disorders.

Histamine intolerance: lack of reproducibility of single symptoms by oral provocation with histamine: A randomised, double-blind, placebo-controlled cross-over study

Komericki P, Klein G, Reider N, Hawranek T, Strimitzer T, Lang R, Kranzelbinder B, Aberer W.

Wien Klin Wochenschr. 2010 Dec 20

OBJECTIVES: The term histamine intolerance stands for a range of symptoms involving various effector organs after the consumption of histamine-rich food. Our intention was to objectify and quantify histamine-associated symptoms and to analyse whether oral administration of the histamine-degrading enzyme diamine oxidase (DAO) caused a reduction of symptoms.

PATIENTS AND METHODS: Four Austrian centres participated. Patients suspected to be histamine intolerant were recruited. The first step consisted in the open oral provocation of these patients with 75 mg of liquid histamine. Patients who developed symptoms were tested in a randomised double blind crossover provocation protocol using histamine-containing and histamine-free tea in combination with DAO capsules or placebo. Main and secondary symptoms (strongest and weaker symptoms based on a ten-point scale) were defined, the grand total of all symptoms of the individual provocation steps was determined and changes in symptoms after administration of DAO were measured.

RESULTS: Thirty nine patients reacted to the open histamine provocation and were enrolled in the blinded part. Here, both the main and secondary symptoms were not reproducible. Subjects reacted sometimes unexpectedly and randomly. Regarding the total symptom scores, the differences between the three treatment groups were statistically significant. The intake of DAO demonstrated a statistically significant reduction of histamine-associated symptoms compared to placebo (P = 0.014).

CONCLUSIONS: Oral provocation with 75 mg of liquid histamine failed to reproduce histamine-associated single symptoms in many patients. One may suggest that histamine-intolerant subjects reacted with different organs on different occasions. As a consequence, reproducibility of single symptoms alone may not be appropriate to diagnose histamine-intolerance whereas a global symptom score could be more appropriate. The fact, that the intake of DAO capsules compared to placebo led to a statistically significant reduction of total symptom scores, may indirectly point in the same direction.

Biogenic amines in foods. Chapter 16
Koutsoumanis K, Tassou C, Nychas GE
Source: Pathogens and Toxins in Foods: Challenges and Interventions, Edited by V.K. Juneja and J.N. Sofos, ASM Press, Washington DC, 2010, ISBN 978-1-55581-459-5, pages 248-274

Effects of a pseudoallergen-free diet on chronic spontaneous urticaria: a prospective trial

Magerl M, Pisarevskaja D, Scheufele R, Zuberbier T, Maurer M.

Source: Allergy. 2010 Jan;65(1):78-83

BACKGROUND: Chronic spontaneous urticaria is a skin disorder that is difficult to manage and can last for years. 'Pseudoallergens' are substances that induce hypersensitive/intolerance reactions that are similar to true allergic reactions. They include food additives, vasoactive substances such as histamine, and some natural substances in fruits, vegetables and spices. Eliminating pseudoallergens from the diet can reduce symptom severity and improve patient quality of life.

AIM: To assess the effects of a pseudoallergen-free diet on disease activity and quality of life in patient's chronic spontaneous urticaria.

METHODS: Study subjects had moderate or severe chronic spontaneous urticaria that had not responded adequately to treatment in primary care. For 3 weeks, subjects followed a pseudoallergen-free diet. They kept a clinical diary, which recorded their wheal and pruritus severity each day, to yield a clinical rating of chronic spontaneous urticaria severity (the UAS4 score). The subjects also completed the DLQI, a validated quality-of-life instrument. Use of antihistamines and glucocorticoids was minimized, recorded, and analysed. Subjects were classified into nine response categories, according to the changes in symptom severity (UAS4), quality of life (DLQI) and medication usage.

RESULTS: From the 140 subjects, there were 20 (14%) strong responders and 19 (14%) partial responders. Additionally, there were nine (6%) subjects who made a substantial reduction in their medication without experiencing worse symptoms or quality of life.

CONCLUSIONS: Altogether the pseudoallergen-free diet is beneficial for one in three patients. The pseudoallergen-free diet is a safe, healthy and cost-free measure to identify patients with chronic spontaneous urticaria that will benefit from avoiding pseudoallergens.

Supplementation of enteric coated Diamine Oxidase improves intestinal degradation of food-born biogenic amines in case of histamine intolerance

Missbichler A, Mayer I, Pongracz C, Gabor F, Komericki P

Clinical Nutrition Supplements (January 2010), 5 (1): 11-11

High concentrations of biogenic amines in food may cause symptoms of histamine intolerance (food intolerance) in persons with reduced activity of Diamine Oxidase (DAO, EC 1.4.3.22) in the lower intestine. DAO is the only enzyme responsible for the degradation of biogenic amines like histamine, putrescine, cadaverine and others in the small intestine. For the use as dietary food the enzyme is purified from biogenic sources, stabilized and processed to small pellets. After enteric coating with shellac, these pellets provide a highly active form of the enzyme directly in the small intestine. Enzymatic activity endures at least 30 min at standardized stomach conditions and is released within 15 min after entering the neutral area of the small intestine to degrade food-borne biogenic amines. DAO degrades histamine, putrescine, cadaverine and other biogenic amines with different affinity, the activity of the enzyme is highly dependent on the concentration of the substrates. This variability in substrate specificity is an important point to be considered in further studies concerning the complex of irritations caused by histamine intolerance. In a double blind, placebo controlled study a statistical significant reduction of symptom score could be shown in patients (n = 39) suffering from food intolerance by supplementation of DAO. Provocation was done with histamine containing tea (75 mg histamine/100 ml tea). Total symptom score was reduced significantly (p = 0.014) in the setting "DAO + histamine" compared to "placebo + histamine". Total symptom score was 10 ± 9; 10 ± 8; 15 ± 9 for the groups DAO + histamine; DAO + tea; placebo + histamine respectively.

IgG-mediated allergy: a new mechanism for migraine attacks?

Pascual J, Oterino A.

Cephalalgia. 2010; 30(7): 777-9

Comment on

Diet restriction in migraine, based on IgG against foods: a clinical double-blind, randomised, cross-over trial. [Cephalalgia. 2010]

Histamine intolerance: a metabolic disease?

Schwelberger H.G.

Inflamm Res. 2010 Mar; 59 Suppl 2:S219-21

OBJECTIVE: To evaluate the evidence regarding the disease concept of histamine intolerance as a state of inadequate histamine inactivation.

METHODS: Keyword-based systematic screening of the scientific literature and of public websites focusing on diagnostic and therapeutic procedures.

RESULTS: Histamine intolerance is commonly diagnosed based solely on subjective reporting of symptoms instead of following systematic diagnostic procedures based on objective laboratory and physical parameters. The only effective long-term therapy is avoidance of histamine-containing food. CONCLUSIONS: The concept of histamine intolerance as a metabolic disease is in need of more experimental and clinical evidence and affected patients will benefit from a clear, evidence-based diagnostic and therapeutic regime.

Polymorphisms of two histamine-metabolizing enzymes genes and childhood allergic asthma: a case control study

Szczepankiewicz A, Bręborowicz A, Sobkowiak P, Popiel A.
Clin Mol Allergy. 2010 Nov 1;8:14
BACKGROUND: Histamine-metabolizing enzymes (N-methyltransferase and amiloride binding protein 1) are responsible for histamine degradation, a biogenic amine involved in allergic inflammation. Genetic variants of HNMT and ABP1 genes were found to be associated with altered enzyme activity. We hypothesized that alleles leading to decreased enzyme activity and, therefore, decreased inactivation of histamine may be responsible for altered susceptibility to asthma.
METHODS: The aim of this study was to analyze polymorphisms within the HNMT and ABP1 genes in the group of 149 asthmatic children and in the group of 156 healthy children. The genetic analysis involved four polymorphisms of the HNMT gene: rs2071048 (-1637T/C), rs11569723 (-411C/T), rs1801105 (Thr105Ile = 314C/T) and rs1050891 (1097A/T) and rs1049793 (His645Asp) polymorphism for ABP1 gene. Genotyping was performed with use of PCR-RFLP. Statistical analysis was performed using Statistica software; linkage disequilibrium analysis was done with use of Haploview software.
RESULTS: We found an association of TT genotype and T allele of Thr105Ile polymorphism of HNMT gene with asthma. For other polymorphisms for HNMT and ABP1 genes, we have not observed relationship with asthma although the statistical power for some SNPs might not have been sufficient to detect an association. In linkage disequilibrium analysis, moderate linkage was found between -1637C/T and -411C/T polymorphisms of HNMT gene. However, no significant differences in haplotype frequencies were found between the group of the patients and the control group.
CONCLUSIONS: Our results indicate modifying influence of histamine N-methyltransferase functional polymorphism on the risk of asthma. The other HNMT polymorphisms and ABP1 functional polymorphism seem unlikely to affect the risk of asthma.

Evaluación del déficit de diaminooxidasa en pacientes con migraña. (Estudio MigraDAO) [Article in Spanish]

Vidal C, Titus F, Guayta-Escolies R
Presentado en la Jornada Internacional de Sensibilización sobre la migraña en el Congreso de Diputados de España, coincidiendo con la presidencia española de la Unión Europea; 24 de mayo de 2010
http://www.dr-healthcare.com/estudio_migradao.pdf

Weinallergien und -intoleranzen

Allergologie, Jahrgang 34, Nr. 8/2011, S. 427–436
Wüthrich B

2009

Histamine pharmacogenomics

García-Martín E, Ayuso P, Martínez C, Blanca M, Agúndez JA
Pharmacogenomics. 2009, 10(5): 867-83
Genetic polymorphisms for histamine-metabolizing enzymes are responsible for interindividual variation in histamine metabolism and are associated with diverse diseases. Initial reports on polymorphisms of histamine-related genes including those coding for the enzymes histidine decarboxylase (HDC), diamine oxidase (ABP1) and histamine N-methyltransferase (HNMT), as well as histamine receptor genes, often have pointed to polymorphisms that occur with extremely low frequencies or that could not be verified by later studies. In contrast, common and functionally significant polymorphisms recently described have been omitted in many association studies. In this review we analyze allele frequencies, functional and clinical impact and interethnic variability on histamine-related polymorphisms. The most relevant nonsynonymous polymorphisms for the HDC gene are rs17740607 Met31Thr, rs16963486 Leu553Phe and rs2073440 Asp644Glu. For ABP1 the most relevant polymorphisms are rs10156191 Thr16Met, rs1049742 Ser332Phe, and particularly because of its functional effect, rs1049793 His645Asp. In addition the ABP1 polymorphisms rs45558339 Ile479Met and rs35070995 His659Asn are relevant to Asian and African subjects, respectively. For HNMT the only nonsynonymous polymorphism present with a relevant frequency is rs1801105 Thr105Ile. For HRH1 the polymorphism rs7651620 Glu270Gly is relevant to African subjects only. The HRH2 rs2067474 polymorphism, located in an enhancer element of the gene

promoter, is common in all populations. No common nonsynonymous SNPs were observed in the HRH3 gene and two SNPs were observed with a significant frequency in the HRH4 gene: rs11665084 Ala138Val and rs11662595 His206Arg. This review summarizes relevant polymorphisms, discusses controversial findings on association of histamine-related polymorphisms and allergies and other diseases, and identifies topics requiring further investigation.

Leserbrief
Source: Allergologie 2009, 32: 41-2
Jarisch R.

Histamine N-methyltransferase 939A>G polymorphism affects mRNA stability in patients with acetylsalicylic acid-intolerant chronic urticaria.
Kim SH, Kang YM, Kim SH, Cho BY, Ye YM, Hur GY, Park HS.
Allergy. 2009 Feb; 64(2):213-21
BACKGROUND: Histamine plays an important role in allergic inflammation. Histamine levels are regulated by histamine N-methyltransferase (HNMT).
OBJECTIVE: To investigate the functional variability of HNMT gene in relation to genetic polymorphisms in patients with aspirin intolerant chronic urticaria (AICU).
METHODS: Two single-nucleotide polymorphisms of the HNMT gene (314C>T, 939A>G) were genotyped in chronic urticaria patients. The functional variability of 3'-untranslated region polymorphism (3'-UTR) was assessed using the pEGFP-HNMT 3'-UTR reporter construct to examine mRNA stability and fluorescence-tagged protein expression. The HNMT enzymatic activities related to the 939A>G polymorphism were examined both in the human mast cells (HMC-1) transfected with the pHNMT CDS-3'-UTR construct and in the patients' red blood cells (RBCs). Histamine release from the basophils of AICU patients was examined.
RESULTS: The 939A>G polymorphism was significantly associated with the AICU phenotype, while no association was found with the 314C>T polymorphism. An in vitro functional study using HMC-1 cells demonstrated that the 939A allele gave lower levels of HNMT mRNA stability, HNMT protein expression, and HNMT enzymatic activity and higher histamine release than the 939G allele. The in vivo functional study demonstrated that the AICU patients with the 939A allele had lower HNMT activity in RBC lysates and higher histamine release from their basophils.
CONCLUSION: The HNMT 939A>G polymorphism lowers HNMT enzymatic activity by decreasing HNMT mRNA stability, which leads to an increase in the histamine level and contributes to the development of AICU.

Diamine oxidase (DAO) serum activity: not a useful marker for diagnosis of histamine intolerance
Kofler H, Aberer W, Deibi M, Hawranek Th, Klein G, Reider N, Fellner N
Allergologie 2009, vol. 32, No. 3, pages 105-109
Although exact numbers on the prevalence of histamine intolerance are lacking, it seems to be on a rise during the last years. The estimated prevalence in the population is 3%. This is particularly true for middle-aged female patients. A deficiency of 1 of the histamine metabolizing enzymes, diamine oxidase (DAO) has been postulated as the main causal factor. Recently, a commercial radioimmunoassay for determination of DAO activity has been launched. To evaluate the clinical impact of this assay for the diagnosis of histamine intolerance, we performed a prospective, multicentre study in 207 adult patients. In 77 patients, a diagnosis of histamine intolerance was made based on clinical criteria, in 67 a diagnosis "in question", and 61 healthy patients without anamnestic evidence for histamine intolerance served as a control. Interestingly, no correlation between diamine oxidase serum levels and clinical status could be found in any of the 3 groups. We, therefore, recommend further investigations, before determination of DAO serum activity should be used as a screening tool for the diagnosis of histamine intolerance.

Analysis of a non-synonymous single nucleotide polymorphism of the human diamine oxidase gene (ref. SNP ID: rs1049793) in patients with Crohn's disease
Lopez P., Agundez J.A., Mendoza J.L., Garcia-Martin E., Martinez C., Fuentes F., Ladero J.M., Taxonera C., Diaz-Rubio M.
Scand J Gastroenterol. 2009;44(10):1207-12
OBJECTIVE: To analyse the possible influence of a non-synonymous single nucleotide polymorphism (SNP) of the histamine-degrading enzyme diamine oxidase (DAO) on genetic susceptibility to Crohn's disease (CD).
MATERIAL AND METHODS: In this prospective, case-control study, 210 unrelated Caucasian consecutive CD patients were recruited at the Inflammatory Bowel Disease Unit of a single tertiary centre (Hospital Clinico San Carlos) in Madrid, Spain. A total of 261 healthy volunteers from the same geographic area were also recruited and matched with patients. Both cases and controls were analysed for the presence of a non-synonymous SNP (rs1049793) of DAO using amplification-restriction procedures of the genotype obtained in a blood sample.

RESULTS: No significant differences were found in the distribution of carriers of the non-synonymous SNP of DAO between CD patients and controls (OR 1.2 (95% CI 0.9-1.6; p=0.3)). Nor were any differences found between carriers and non-carriers of the non-synonymous SNP in demographic characteristics, phenotypes, complications or treatment of CD.

CONCLUSIONS: The study of a non-synonymous SNP (rs1049793) of DAO does not seem to be of use in assessing susceptibility to CD, either as a marker of disease activity or as a marker of clinical behaviour in patients with the disease.

The structure and inhibition of human diamine oxidase

McGrath AP, Hilmer KM, Collyer CA, Shepard EM, Elmore BO, Brown DE, Dooley DM, Guss JM
Biochemistry. 2009 Oct 20;48(41):9810-22

Humans have three functioning genes that encode copper-containing amine oxidases. The product of the AOC1 gene is a so-called diamine oxidase (hDAO), named for its substrate preference for diamines, particularly histamine. hDAO has been cloned and expressed in insect cells and the structure of the native enzyme determined by X-ray crystallography to a resolution of 1.8 A. The homodimeric structure has the archetypal amine oxidase fold. Two active sites, one in each subunit, are characterized by the presence of a copper ion and a topaquinone residue formed by the post-translational modification of a tyrosine. Although hDAO shares 37.9% sequence identity with another human copper amine oxidase, semicarbazide sensitive amine oxidase or vascular adhesion protein-1, its substrate binding pocket and entry channel are distinctly different in accord with the different substrate specificities. The structures of two inhibitor complexes of hDAO, berenil and pentamidine, have been refined to resolutions of 2.1 and 2.2 A, respectively. They bind noncovalently in the active-site channel. The inhibitor binding suggests that an aspartic acid residue, conserved in all diamine oxidases but absent from other amine oxidases, is responsible for the diamine specificity by interacting with the second amino group of preferred diamine substrates.

Hypertensive crisis and cheese

Rao T.S.S and Yeragani VK
Indian J Psychiatry. 2009; 51(1): 65–66

Histamine intolerance: overestimated or underestimated?

Schwelberger HG.
Praxis (Bern 1994). 2009; 98(7): 375-87

[Histamine intolerance mimics anorexia nervosa.] [Article in German]

Stolze I, Peters KP, Herbst RA.
Hautarzt. 2009 Nov 13

Histamine intolerance is a clinically heterogeneous disease. We present a woman who suffered from weight loss, diarrhea, abdominal pain, headache, flushing and bronchial asthma for several years. When placed on a histamine-poor diet, she experienced weight gain and improvement of other all signs and symptoms, supporting the diagnosis of histamine intolerance. Therefore, this disease should be included in the differential diagnosis of anorexia nervosa.

Foods and supplements in the management of migraine headaches

Sun-Edelstein C, Mauskop A
Clin J Pain. 2009; 25(5): 446-52

OBJECTIVE: Although a wide range of acute and preventative medications are now available for the treatment of migraine headaches, many patients will not have a significant improvement in the frequency and severity of their headaches unless lifestyle modifications are made. Also, given the myriad side effects of traditional prescription medications, there is an increasing demand for "natural" treatment like vitamins and supplements for common ailments such as headaches. Here, we discuss the role of food triggers in the management of migraines, and review the evidence for supplements in migraine treatment.

METHODS: A review of the English language literature on preclinical and clinical studies of any type on food triggers, vitamins, supplements, and migraine headaches was conducted.

RESULTS: A detailed nutritional history is helpful in identifying food triggers. Although the data surrounding the role of certain foods and substances in triggering headaches is controversial, certain subsets of patients may be sensitive to phenylethylamine, tyramine, aspartame, monosodium glutamate, nitrates, nitrites, alcohol, and caffeine. The available evidence for the efficacy of certain vitamins and supplements in preventing migraines supports the use of these agents in the migraine treatment.

CONCLUSIONS: The identification of food triggers, with the help of food diaries, is an inexpensive way to reduce migraine headaches. We also recommend the use of the following supplements in the preventative treatment of migraines, in decreasing order of preference: magnesium, Petasites hybridus, feverfew, coenzyme Q10, riboflavin, and alpha lipoic acid.

Exogenous histamine aggravates eczema in a subgroup of patients with atopic dermatitis
Worm M, Fiedler EM, Dölle S, Schink T, Hemmer W, Jarisch R, Zuberbier T.
Acta Derm Venerol 2009; 89: 52–6

Food and beverages may contain high amounts of histamine and thus may cause symptoms after ingestion. The aim of this study was to investigate the role of ingested histamine in atopic dermatitis. Patients with atopic dermatitis had to maintain a histamine-free diet for one week. Consecutively, double-blind, placebo-controlled provocations were performed with histamine-hydrochloride and placebo. The clinical outcome was assessed by determination of the SCORAD. Before and 30 min after each provocation blood was collected for measurement of plasma histamine levels and diamine oxidase activity. Thirty-six patients with atopic dermatitis completed the diet. Twelve of 36 showed a significant improvement of the SCORAD after one week of the diet. After provocation tests 11 of 36 showed aggravation of eczema. Plasma histamine was significantly higher in patients with atopic dermatitis compared with controls (p>< 0.001), whereas diamine oxidase activity was similar in both groups. Our data indicate that ingestion of moderate or high amounts of histamine-hydrochloride may aggravate eczema in a subgroup of patients with atopic dermatitis. Plasma histamine and diamine oxidase activity were not associated with the clinical response to histamine.

[Food allergy, food intolerance or functional disorder?] [Article in German]
Wüthrich B.
Inflamm Res. 2009 Apr; 58 Suppl 1:51-2

The term "food allergy" is widely misused for all sorts of symptoms and diseases caused by food. Food allergy (FA) is an adverse reaction to food (food hypersensitivity) occurring in susceptible individuals, which is mediated by a classical immune mechanism specific for the food itself. The best established mechanism in FA is due to the presence of IgE antibodies against the offending food. Food intolerance (FI) are all non-immune-mediated adverse reactions to food. The subgroups of FI are enzymatic (e.g. lactose intolerance due to lactase deficiency), pharmacological (reactions against biogenic amines, histamine intolerance), and undefined food intolerance (e.g. against some food additives). The diagnosis of an IgE-mediated FA is made by a carefully taken case history, supported by the demonstration of an IgE sensitization either by skin prick tests or by in vitro tests, and confirmed by positive oral provocation. For scientific purposes the only accepted test for the confirmation of FA/FI is a properly performed double-blind, placebo-controlled food challenge (DBPCFC). A panel of recombinant allergens, produced as single allergenic molecules, may in future improve the diagnosis of IgE-mediated FA. Due to a lack of causal treatment possibilities, the elimination of the culprit "food allergen" from the diet is the only therapeutic option for patients with real food allergy.

2008

Nonsynonymous polymorphisms of histamine-metabolising enzymes in patients with Parkinson's disease
Agúndez JA, Luengo A, Herráez O, Martínez C, Alonso-Navarro H, Jiménez-Jiménez FJ, García-Martín E
Neuromolecular Med. 2008; 10(1): 10-6

OBJECTIVE: To analyze genetically based impairment in histamine-metabolising enzymes in patients with Parkinson's disease (PD).
METHODS: Leukocytary DNA from 214 PD patients and a control group of 295 unrelated healthy individuals was studied for nonsynonymous histamine N-methyltransferase (HNMT) and diamine oxidase (ABP1) polymorphisms by using amplification-restriction analyses.
RESULTS: An association of the HNMT Thr105Ile polymorphism, but not of the ABP1 His645Asp polymorphism, with PD was observed. Patients with PD showed a higher frequency of homozygous HNMT genotypes leading to high activity with a gene-dose effect (P < 0.001), as compared to healthy subjects. These findings were independent of gender, but the association with the HNMT polymorphism is higher among patients with late-onset PD (P < 0.0001).
CONCLUSION: These results, combined with previous findings indicating alterations in histamine levels in patients with PD, suggest that alterations of histamine homeostasis in the SNC are associated with the risk for PD.

[Histamine intolerance syndrome. Its significance for ENT medicine] [Article in German]
Böttcher I, Klimek L.
HNO. 2008 Aug; 56(8):776-83

The symptoms of histamine intolerance are similar to those of the IgE-mediated allergic immune response. Patients affected by this disease, mostly middle-aged women, suffer from conditions such as headaches and rhinitis, particularly after consuming histamine-rich foods, indulging in alcoholic beverages, or taking certain pharmaceuticals. Moreover, life-threatening anaphylactic reactions can be observed with this syndrome. This article describes the biochemical processes and cellular background of histamine intolerance syndrome and discusses the diagnostic and therapeutic procedures within otorhinolaryngology. It is our goal to direct attention to this often unrecognized clinical picture and to contribute to increased immunologic knowledge of this disease.

[Intolerance to food additives: an update] [Article in Italian]

Cardinale F, Mangini F, Berardi M, Sterpeta Loffredo M, Chinellato I, Dellino A, Cristofori F, Di Domenico F, Mastrototaro MF, Cappiello A, Centoducati T, Carella F, Armenio L.

Minerva Pediatr. 2008 Dec; 60(6):1401-9

Contrary to common believing, the prevalence of the intolerance to food additives in the general population is rather low. Nowadays many doubts persist with regard both to the pathogenetic mechanisms and to the clinical and diagnostic aspects in this field. Symptoms due to, or exacerbated from, food additives usually involve non-IgE-mediate mechanisms (pseudo-allergic reactions, PAR) and are usually less severe of those induced by food allergy. The most frequent clinical feature of the intolerance to food additives still remains the urticaria-angioedema syndrome, although these substances are really involved only in a minority of patients. Other possible clinical features include anaphylaxis, atopic eczema, behaviour disturbances, asthma and non-allergic rhinitis. The diagnostic approach consists in diary cards, reporting symptoms and food habits, elimination diet and double blinded placebo-controlled oral challenge with suspected additives. However, such procedure still remains poorly standardized and numerous uncertainties persist with regard to optimal conditions for performing and interpret the challenge results. The therapeutic approach consists in the exclusion of foods and products containing the additive involved, and, in patients not compliant to the diet, in treatment with symptomatic drugs.

European Commission (2008)

COMMISSION REGULATION (EC) No 889/2008 of 5 September 2008

laying down detailed rules for the implementation of Council Regulation (EC) No 834/2007 on organic production and labelling of organic products with regard to organic production, labelling and control

Histamine-N-Methyl Transferase Polymorphism and Risk for Migraine

García-Martín E, Martínez C, Serrador M, Alonso-Navarro H, Navacerrada F, Agúndez JAG, Jiménez-Jiménez FJ

Headache: The Journal of Head and Face Pain, 2008, 48/9, 1343–1348

BACKGROUND/OBJECTIVES: Histamine has been implicated in the pathogenesis of migraine. In the CNS, histamine is almost exclusively metabolized by the polymorphic enzyme histamine N-methyltransferase (HNMT). The HNMT gene (chromosome 2q22.1), shows diverse single nucleotide polymorphisms. One of these, located in exon 4 C314T, causes the amino acid substitution Thr105Ile, related to decreased enzyme activity. The aim of this study was to investigate the possible association between HNMT polymorphism and the risk for migraine.

METHODS: We studied the frequency of the HNMT genotypes and allelic variantes in 197 patients with migraine and 245 healthy controls using a PCR-RLFP method.

RESULTS: The frequencies of the HNMT genotypes and allelic variants did not differ significantly between migraine patients and controls, and were unrelated with the age of onset of migraine attacks, gender, personal history of allergic diseases, family history of migraine, or presence of aura.

CONCLUSIONS: The results of the present study suggest that HNMT polymorphism in not related with the risk for migraine.

NOTE: *"We studied 197 unselected and unrelated patients with diagnostic criteria for migraine according with classification of the International Headache Society who did not fulfilled criteria for other headache types"*

Plasma histamine levels and symptoms in double blind placebo controlled histamine provocation

Giera B, Straube S, Konturek P, Hahn EG, Raithel M.

Inflamm Res 2008; 57: 1–2

Histamine intolerance (Hi) is known as a misbalance between histamine (H) present in the body and H degrading enzymes (i.e. diamine oxidase, histamine N-methyltransferase. To establish a method for the diagnosis of Hi, double blind placebo controlled oral H provocation was performed. Diagnosis of Hi was defined as confirmed (corresponding to the recent literature) when there was a rise of plasma H level of at least 40% compared to pre-test H concentration together with at least one subjective or objective symptom.

Case-control cohort study of patients' perceptions of disability in mastocytosis

Hermine O, Lortholary O, Leventhal PS, Catteau A, Soppelsa F, Baude C, Cohen-Akenine A, Palmérini F, Hanssens K, Yang Y, Sobol H, Fraytag S, Ghez D, Suarez F, Barete S, Casassus P, Sans B, Arock M, Kinet JP, Dubreuil P, Moussy A.

PLoS One. 2008 May 28; 3(5): e2266

BACKGROUND: Indolent forms of mastocytosis account for more than 90% of all cases, but the types and type and severity of symptoms and their impact on the quality of life have not been well studied.

We therefore performed a case-control cohort study to examine self-reported disability and impact of symptoms on the quality of life in patients with mastocytosis.

METHODOLOGY/PRINCIPAL FINDINGS: In 2004, 363 mastocytosis patients and 90 controls in France were asked to rate to their overall disability (OPA score) and the severity of 38 individual symptoms. The latter was used to calculate a composite score (AFIRMM score). Of the 363 respondents, 262 were part of an ongoing pathophysiological study so that the following data were available: World Health Organization classification, standard measures of physical and psychological disability, existence of the D816V KIT mutation, and serum tryptase level. The mean OPA and AFIRMM scores and the standard measures of disability indicated that most mastocytosis patients suffer from disabilities due to the disease. Surprisingly, the patient's measurable and perceived disabilities did not differ according to disease classification or presence or absence of the D816V KIT mutation or an elevated (> or = 20 ng/mL) serum tryptase level. Also, 32 of the 38 AFIRMM symptoms were more common in patients than controls, but there were not substantial differences according to disease classification, presence of the D816V mutation, or the serum tryptase level.

CONCLUSIONS: On the basis of these results and for the purposes of treatment, we propose that mastocytosis be first classified as aggressive or indolent and that indolent mastocytosis then be categorized according to the severity of patients' perceived symptoms and their impact on the quality of life. In addition, it appears that mastocytosis patients suffer from more symptoms and greater disability than previously thought, that mastocytosis may therefore be under-diagnosed, and that the symptoms of the indolent forms of mastocytosis might be due more to systemic release of mediators than mast cell burden.

C314T polymorphism in histamine N-methyltransferase gene and susceptibility to duodenal ulcer in Chinese population
Hailong C, Mei Q, Zhang L, Xu J.
Clin Chim Acta. 2008; 389(1-2): 51-4
Erratum in
Clin Chim Acta. 2008 May;391(1-2):130. Cao, Haillong [corrected to Cao, Hailong].
BACKGROUND: Histamine is a regulator of gastric acid secretion, which is involved in the development of duodenal ulcer (DU). Histamine is metabolized by both histamine N-methyltransferase (HNMT) and diamine oxidase, and its local action is terminated primarily by methylation which is catalyzed by HNMT.
METHODS: Polymerase chain reaction-restriction fragment length polymorphism assay was used to identify the polymorphism of the point mutation C314T of HNMT gene of 498 Chinese patients with DU and 151 healthy individuals.
RESULTS: In normal controls, the allele frequency of HNMT T314 was 3.3%, which was significantly lower than American Caucasians. The HNMT T314 allele was detected in 3.5% of the DU patients. In cases and controls, the frequency of C/C genotypes were 93.0% and 93.4%, respectively. The HNMT T/T genotype was not found in this population. No significant differences were seen in both genotype frequencies and allele frequencies between DU groups and controls. After stratified by H. pylori infection, they also could not reach significant differences in our current study.
CONCLUSION: The HNMT T314 allele frequency is lower in Chinese population than in American Caucasians. No association can be found in the involvement of HNMT C314T polymorphism in the susceptibility to duodenal ulcer.

Association of the histamine N-methyltransferase C314T (Thr105Ile) polymorphism with atopic dermatitis in Caucasian children
Kennedy MJ, Loehle JA, Griffin AR, Doll MA, Kearns GL, Sullivan JE, Hein DW.
Pharmacotherapy. 2008, 28(12): 1495-501
STUDY OBJECTIVE: To investigate potential associations between the histamine N-methyltransferase (HNMT) gene, HNMT, C314T (Thr105Ile) polymorphism and atopic dermatitis in a cohort of Caucasian children.
DESIGN: Prospective, multicenter, genotype-association study.
SETTING: Four academic, tertiary care medical centers within the Pediatric Pharmacology Research Unit network.
PARTICIPANTS: Two hundred forty-nine Caucasian children aged 6 months-5 years with atopic dermatitis (127 patients) or without (122 control subjects).
INTERVENTION: Buccal swabs (one swab/cheek) were performed to obtain epithelial cells for extraction of genomic DNA.
MEASUREMENTS AND MAIN RESULTS: Data were collected on severity of atopic dermatitis, oral antihistamine treatment, and treatment response through parental report. The HNMT genotypes were successfully obtained in 116 control subjects and 122 patients with atopic dermatitis. Frequencies of the T314 variant allele (0.12 vs 0.06, p=0.04) and combined CT/TT genotype (0.24 vs 0.12, p=0.02) were significantly higher in children with atopic dermatitis compared with control subjects. Children with genotypes conferring reduced HNMT activity were 2 times more likely to have atopic dermatitis than those who were homozygous for the C314 reference allele.

CONCLUSION: Increased histamine levels in patients with atopic dermatitis may result, at least in part, from reduced enzymatic inactivation via HNMT. Genetically associated reduction in histamine biotransformation may therefore contribute to the pathogenesis, persistence, and progression of atopic dermatitis. If confirmed, these data indicate that HNMT genotype might represent a common risk factor for development of atopic dermatitis, asthma, and allergic rhinitis and may be useful in identifying individuals who are candidates for early preventive pharmacotherapeutic intervention. Additional longitudinal studies will be required to assess the relationship between genotype, disease severity, and antihistamine response.

Oral verabreichte Diaminoxidase (DAO) bei Patienten mit Verdacht auf Histamin-Intoleranz
Komericki P, Klein G, Hawranek T, Land R, Reider N, Stri-mitzer T, Kranzelbinder B, Aberer W.
Allergologie 2008; 31: 190

Both catabolic pathways of histamine via histamine-N-methyl-transferase and diamine oxidase are diminished in colonic mucosa of patients with food allergy
Kuefner MA, Schwelberger HG, Weidenhiller M, Hahn EG, Raithel M.
Inflamm Res 2004; 53: 31–2

The nonsynonymous Thr105Ile polymorphism of the histamine N-methyltransferase is associated to the risk of developing essential tremor
Ledesma MC, García-Martín E, Alonso-Navarro H, Martínez C, Jiménez-Jiménez FJ, Benito-León J, Puertas I, Rubio L, López-Alburquerque T, Agúndez JA
Neuromolecular Med. 2008;10(4): 356-61
OBJECTIVE: We analyzed in patients with essential tremor (ET) the Thr105Ile polymorphism of the Histamine N-methyltransferase (HNMT) enzyme that is associated to Parkinson's disease (PD) risk.
METHODS: Leukocytary DNA from 204 ET patients and a control group of 295 unrelated healthy individuals was studied for the nonsynonymous HNMT Thr105Ile polymorphism by using amplification-restriction analyses.
RESULTS: Patients with ET showed a higher frequency of homozygous HNMT 105Thr genotypes leading to high metabolic activity ($p < 0.015$) with a statistically significant gene-dose effect, as compared to healthy subjects. These findings were independent of gender, and of tremor localization, but the association of the HNMT polymorphism is more prominent among patients with late-onset ET ($p < 0.007$).
CONCLUSION: These results, combined with previous findings indicating alterations in the frequency for the HNMT Thr105Ile polymorphism in patients with PD, suggest that alterations of histamine homeostasis in the SNC are associated with the risk of movement disorders.

Effects of histamine and diamine oxidase activities on pregnancy: a critical review.
Maintz L, Schwarzer V, Bieber T, van der Ven K, Novak N.
Hum Reprod Update. 2008 Sep-Oct; 14(5):485-95
BACKGROUND: Histamine has been assumed to contribute to embryo-uterine interactions due to its vasoactive, differentiation and growth-promoting properties. However, its exact functions in pregnancy are unclear. The histamine-degrading enzyme diamine oxidase (DAO) is produced in high amounts by the placenta and has been supposed to act as a metabolic barrier to prevent excessive entry of bioactive histamine from the placenta into the maternal or fetal circulation.
METHODS: The literature available on PubMed published in English between 1910 and 2008 has been searched using the isolated and combined key words histamine, diamine oxidase, pregnancy, placenta, endometrium, miscarriage, implantation, pre-eclampsia, intrauterine growth retardation, diabetes and embryonic histamine-releasing factor (EHRF).
RESULTS: High expression of the histamine-producing enzyme histidine decarboxylase in the placenta, histamine receptors at the feto-maternal interface and the existence of an EHRF suggest a physiological role of histamine during gestation. The balance between histamine and DAO seems to be crucial for an uncomplicated course of pregnancy. Reduced DAO activities have been found in multiple heterogeneous complications of pregnancy such as diabetes, threatened and missed abortion and trophoblastic disorders. Whether women with histamine intolerance suffer from more complicated pregnancies and higher abortion rates due to impaired DAO activities and if low DAO levels or genetic modifications in the DAO gene might therefore represent a prognostic factor for a higher risk of abortion, has not been investigated yet.
CONCLUSIONS: Low activities of the histamine-degrading enzyme DAO might indicate high-risk pregnancies, although high intra- and interindividual variations limit its value as a screening tool.

Oxidative stability of tree nut oils
Miraliakbari H, Shahidi F
J Agric Food Chem. 2008; 56(12): 4751-9
The oxidative stability of selected tree nut oils was examined. The oils of almond, Brazil nut, hazelnut, pecan, pine nut, pistachio, and walnut were extracted using two solvent extraction systems, namely,

hexane and chloroform/methanol. The chloroform/methanol system afforded a higher oil yield for each tree nut type examined (pine nut had the highest oil content, whereas almond had the lowest). The fatty acid compositions of tree nut oils were analyzed using gas chromatography, showing that oleic acid was the predominant fatty acid in all samples except pine nut and walnut oils, which contained high amounts of linoleic acid. The tocopherol compositions were analyzed using high-performance liquid chromatography, showing that alpha- and gamma-tocopherols were the predominant tocopherol homologues present; however delta- and beta-tocopherols were also detected in some samples. The oxidative stability of nonstripped and stripped tree nut oils was examined under two conditions, namely, accelerated autoxidation and photooxidation. Progression of oxidation was monitored using tests for conjugated dienes, peroxide value, p-anisidine value, and headspace volatiles. Primary products of oxidation persisted in the earlier stages of oxidation, whereas secondary oxidation product levels increased dramatically during the later stages of oxidation. Hexanal was the major headspace aldehyde formed in all oxidized samples except walnut oil, which contained primarily propanal. Results showed that chloroform/methanol-extracted oils were more stable than hexane-extracted oils in both the accelerated autoxidation and photooxidation studies. Oils of pecan and pistachio were the most stable, whereas oils of pine nut and walnut were the least stable.

The histamine N-methyltransferase T105I polymorphism affects active site structure and dynamics
Rutherford K, Parson WW, Daggett V.
Biochemistry. 2008; 47(3): 893-901
Histamine N-methyltransferase (HNMT) is the primary enzyme responsible for inactivating histamine in the mammalian brain. The human HNMT gene contains a common threonine-isoleucine polymorphism at residue 105, distal from the active site. The 105I variant has decreased activity and lower protein levels than the 105T protein. Crystal structures of both variants have been determined but reveal little regarding how the T105I polymorphism affects activity. We performed molecular dynamics simulations for both 105T and 105I at 37 degrees C to explore the structural and dynamic consequences of the polymorphism. The simulations indicate that replacing Thr with the larger Ile residue leads to greater burial of residue 105 and heightened intramolecular interactions between residue 105 and residues within helix alpha3 and strand beta3. This altered, tighter packing is translated to the active site, resulting in the reorientation of several cosubstrate-binding residues. The simulations also show that the hydrophobic histamine-binding domain in both proteins undergoes a large-scale breathing motion that exposes key catalytic residues and lowers the hydrophobicity of the substrate-binding site.

[Histamine intolerance: Is the determination of diamine oxidase activity in the serum useful in routine clinical practice?]
Histaminintoleranz: Wie sinn voll ist die Bestimmung der Diaminoxidase-Aktivitätim Serum in der all täglichen klinischen Praxis?
Töndury B, Wüthrich B, Schmid-Grendeleier P, Seifert B, Ballmer-Weber B.
Allergologie. 2008; 31: 350-356
BACKGROUND: An intolerance to food might be induced by an impaired enzymatic histamine degradation due to a deficiency of diamine oxidase (DAO) activity (Histamine intolerance [HIT]).
OBJECTIVE: The aim of the study was to investigate if patients histories, that are suggestive to HIT have a significant reduced serum DAO activity compared to patients without history of HIT.
METHODS: 61 patients and 20 controls were studied. 26 patients (strong HIT) had a history of at least two typical symptoms of HIT with relation to the intake of at least two histamine rich foods. 35 patients (moderate HIT) had a history of at least one symptom after the intake of at least one hista mine rich food (but not both). 20 healthy volunteers (conrol) did not have any symptoms of HIT. Patients were interviewed on type of clinical symptoms and the relation of symptoms to food in gestion. Sera were analysed for DAO activity by an ELISA test.
RESULTS: No difference of serum DAO levels could be found between groups of dif ferent history of HIT.
CONCLUSION: Based on the patients history with allergy like symptoms occurring with intake of histamine rich food, determination of DAO activity in the serum does not facilitate diagnosis of HIT in routine clinical practice

2007

Endometriosis, dysmenorrhea and diet--what is the evidence?
Fjerbaek A, Knudsen UB.
Eur J Obstet Gynecol Reprod Biol. 2007 Jun;132(2):140-7
The objective of this study is to assess the literature concerning the effect of diet on endometriosis and dysmenorrhea and to elucidate evidential support, to give dietary recommendations to women suffering from these conditions. A systematic search in electronic databases on a relationship between diet and endometriosis/dysmenorrhea was performed. Data on diet and endometriosis were limited to four trials of which two were animal studies. The articles concerning human consumption found some

relation between disease and low intake of vegetable and fruit and high intake of vegetarian polyunsaturated fat, ham, beef and other red meat. Results concerning fish intake were not consistent. Eight trials of different design, with a total of 1097 women, investigated the relationship between diet and dysmenorrhea. Intake of fish oil seemed to have a positive effect on pain symptoms. This study concludes that literature on diet and endometriosis is sparse, whereas eight studies have looked at diet and dysmenorrhea. No clear recommendations on what diet to eat or refrain from to reduce the symptoms of endometriosis can be given, while a few studies indicate that fish oil can reduce dysmenorrhea. Further research is recommended on both subjects.

Histamine in food: is there anything to worry about?

W.A. Fogel WA, Lewinski A, Jochem J
Biochemical Society Transactions (2007) 35, 349–352

Biogenic mono-, di- and poly-amines are widely distributed among living organisms. The amines fulfil many important functions in the human body both in the periphery and brain. Some authors suggest that foods rich in biogenic amines, especially histamine, present high health hazards for consumers. However, this is conditional on a range of other factors. The alimentary tract is well equipped with enzymes that inactivate amines and the blood–brain barrier prevents them entering the brain from the circulation. Oxidative deamination, methylation, acetylation and transglutamylation are the degradation pathways which operate efficiently in the stomach, intestines and liver. Particularly important is oxidative deamination. Food histamine poisoning or cheese reaction, manifested itself in patients treated with drugs that inhibit amine oxidases or in patients showing an enterocytic diamine oxidase deficit. It is rather food allergy, which should worry us more, as endogenous histamine release from mast cells is more dangerous. Preventive measures should be undertaken against increases in food allergies.

Polymorphisms of histamine-metabolizing enzymes and clinical manifestations of asthma and allergic rhinitis

García-Martín E, García-Menaya J, Sánchez B, Martínez C, Rosendo R, Agúndez JA
Clin Exp Allergy. 2007; 37(8): 1175-82

BACKGROUND: Polymorphisms of enzymes involved in histamine biodisposition may affect clinical symptoms in diseases related to histamine, such as asthma or allergic rhinitis (AR).
OBJECTIVE: This study aims to analyse two common polymorphisms in genes coding for histamine-metabolizing enzymes in patients with allergic diseases.
METHODS: Five-hundred and sixty-five individuals participated in the study, including 270 unrelated patients with asthma and/or AR recruited from a single centre and 295 healthy volunteers. Participants were analysed for the presence of Thr105Ile and His645Asp amino acid substitutions at histamine N-methyltransferase (HNMT) and diamine oxidase (amiloride binding protein 1) enzymes, respectively, by amplification-restriction procedures.
RESULTS: The variant HNMT allele frequencies were slightly higher among patients with asthma [16.0%, 95% confidence interval (CI) 12.0-20.0] and among patients with rhinitis (13.2, 95% CI 10.3-16.1) as compared with healthy subjects (11.5 95% CI 8.9-14.1). The variant ABP1 allele frequencies were similar among patients with asthma (30.8%, 95% CI 25.7-35.9), rhinitis (28.7, 95% CI 24.8-32.6) and healthy subjects (26.8 95% CI 23.2-30.3). Individuals carrying mutated ABP1 alleles presented allergy symptoms with significantly lower IgE levels as compared with individuals without mutated genes, with a significant gene-dose effect (P<0.001). In addition, the percentage of individuals presenting symptoms without eosinophilia was significantly higher among homozygous carriers of ABP1 variant alleles (P<0.020) as compared with the rest of the atopic patients.
CONCLUSION: There is a lack of association between the allelic variants studied and the risk of developing allergic asthma and rhinitis. However, patients carrying the His645Asp polymorphism of ABP1 are more prone to developing symptoms with lower IgE levels.

Histamine and histamine intolerance.

Maintz L, Novak N.
Am J Clin Nutr 2007; 85: 1185–96

Histamine and histamine intolerance.

Maintz L, Novak N.
Dtsch Med Wochenschr. 2007 Oct;132(40):p21

Histamine intolerance results from a disequilibrium of accumulated histamine and the capacity for histamine degradation. Histamine is a biogenic amine that occurs to various degrees in many foods. In healthy persons, dietary histamine can be rapidly detoxified by amine oxidases, whereas persons with low amine oxidase activity are at risk of histamine toxicity. Diamine oxidase (DAO) is the main enzyme for the metabolism of ingested histamine. It has been proposed that DAO, when functioning as a secretory protein, may be responsible for scavenging extracellular histamine after mediator release. Conversely, histamine N-methyltransferase, the other important enzyme inactivating histamine, is a cytosolic protein that can convert histamine only in the intracellular space of cells. An impaired histamine degradation based on reduced DAO activity and the resulting histamine excess may cause numerous symptoms mimicking an allergic reaction. The ingestion of histamine-rich food or of alcohol or drugs that release histamine or block DAO may provoke diarrhea, headache, rhinoconjunctival symptoms, asthma, hypotension, arrhythmia, urticaria, pruritus, flushing, and other conditions in patients with histamine intolerance. Symptoms can be reduced by a histamine-free diet or be eliminated by antihistamines. However, because of the multifaceted nature of the symptoms, the existence of histamine intolerance has been underestimated, and further studies based on double-blind, placebo-controlled provocations are needed. In patients in whom the abovementioned symptoms are triggered by the corresponding substances and who have a negative diagnosis of allergy or internal disorders, histamine intolerance should be considered as an underlying pathomechanism.

Potato lectin activates basophils and mast cells of atopic subjects by its interaction with core chitobiose of cell-bound non-specific immunoglobulin E
Pramod SN, Venkatesh YP, Mahesh PA
Clin Exp Immunol. 2007; 148(3): 391–401
A major factor in non-allergic food hypersensitivity could be the interaction of dietary lectins with mast cells and basophils. Because immunoglobulin E (IgE) contains 10–12% carbohydrates, lectins can activate and degranulate these cells by cross-linking the glycans of cell-bound IgE. The present objective focuses on the effect of potato lectin (Solanum tuberosum agglutinin; STA) for its ability to release histamine from basophils in vitro and mast cells in vivo from non-atopic and atopic subjects. In this study, subjects were selected randomly based on case history and skin prick test responses with food, pollen and house dust mite extracts. Skin prick test (SPT) was performed with STA at 100 µg/ml concentration. Histamine release was performed using leucocytes from non-atopic and atopic subjects and rat peritoneal exudate cells. SPT on 110 atopic subjects using STA showed 39 subjects positive (35%); however, none showed STA-specific IgE; among 20 non-atopic subjects, none were positive by SPT. Maximal histamine release was found to be 65% in atopic subjects (n = 7) compared to 28% in non-atopic subjects (n = 5); the release was inhibited specifically by oligomers of N-acetylglucosamine and correlates well with serum total IgE levels (R2 = 0·923). Binding of STA to N-linked glycoproteins (horseradish peroxidase, avidin and IgG) was positive by dot blot and binding assay. As potato lectin activates and degranulates both mast cells and basophils by interacting with the chitobiose core of IgE glycans, higher intake of potato may increase the clinical symptoms as a result of non-allergic food hypersensitivity in atopic subjects.

Amitriptyline affects histamine-N-methyltransferase and diamine oxidase activity in rats and guinea pigs
Rajtar S, Irman-Florjanc T.
Eur J Pharmacol. 2007 Nov 28;574(2-3):201-8
Histamine participates in numerous physiological and patophysiological processes. Drugs which interfere with the histamine actions are antagonists and agonists of histamine receptors. Histamine degrading enzymes as a possible target for modifying histamine action have so far not been extensively studied. Therefore we examined in vivo and in vitro effects of amitriptyline on two histamine degrading enzymes - diamine oxidase and histamine-N-methyltransferase. We were interested in the in vivo effects of amitriptyline on the diamine oxidase release into guinea pig plasma after heparin stimulation and in effects on the activity and gene expression of both histamine degrading enzymes in different guinea pig tissues. Amitriptyline's in vitro effects on the diamine oxidase and histamine-N-methyltransferase activities were measured in guinea pig and also in rat. Enzyme activities were determined with the radiometric micro-assay. The results showed that amitriptyline in vivo changed the profile of the heparin-induced diamine oxidase release, which could be due to changes in at least three processes: diamine oxidase release into plasma, protein synthesis and enzyme activity at the molecular level. Amitriptyline in some tissues (lung and spleen) amplified the mRNA expression of histamine degrading enzymes. Furthermore, the activities of these enzymes were increased in most examined tissues of amitriptyline treated guinea pigs. In vitro studies indicate that amitriptyline differently affects diamine oxidase and histamine-N-methyltransferase in two different rodent species, guinea pig and rat. Our study proved that amitriptyline enhances the histamine degrading processes in guinea pig, what might importantly contribute to lower histamine levels.

Association of THR105Ile, a functional polymorphism of histamine N-methyltransferase (HNMT), with alcoholism in German Caucasians.
Reuter M, Jeste N, Klein T, Hennig J, Goldman D, Enoch MA, Oroszi G
Drug Alcohol Depend. 2007; 87(1): 69-75
BACKGROUND: CNS histamine has been shown to have an inhibitory effect on reward and it is implicated in the etiology of addiction and stress. Histamine N-methyltransferase (HNMT) is believed to be the sole pathway for termination of the neurotransmitter action of histamine in mammalian brain. A common, functional polymorphism, a C314T transition in the HNMT gene, results in a

Thr105Ile substitution of the protein encoded. A recent study has shown that the frequency of the Ile105 allele was significantly lower in alcoholics compared to that in non-alcoholics in Finns and Plains American Indians. Following up these results, we tested whether the Thr105Ile polymorphism was associated with alcoholism in German Caucasians.

METHODS: Thr105Ile was genotyped in n=366 psychiatrically interviewed German Caucasian ICD-10 lifetime alcoholics, along with n=200 ethnically matched controls.

RESULTS: No significant difference was found in the frequency of the Ile105 allele between alcoholics (0.11) and controls (0.10) (chi(2)=0.21, d.f.=1, p=0.647). Likewise, genotype distributions did not differ significantly. However, the frequency of the Ile105 allele was significantly lower in male alcoholics with a family history of alcoholism compared to that in male alcoholics without a family history of alcoholism (chi(2)=4.07, d.f.=1, p=0.044).

CONCLUSIONS: In German Caucasians the association of the HNMT Thr105Ile polymorphism with alcoholism was not replicated per se, but a congruent association was found between the Ile105 allele and family history of alcoholism supporting the protective role of the Ile105 allele against alcoholism.

Biogene Amine – Ernährung bei Histamin-Intoleranz

Steneberg A

Umwelt & Gesundheit 2/2007: 47-56

Non-allergic reactions to food are often defined to be induced by biogenic amines (e.g. histamine), corresponding to symp-toms like headache, rhinitis, respiratory, digestive complaints and eczema. The extent of Histamine intolerance (HIT) has possibly been underestimated. HIT is the consequence of histamine rich nutrition and less important related to the histamine release from mediator cells like mast cells (MC), mucose mast cells (MMC) and basophil granulocytes
in high developed species. Histamine and other biogenic amines are produced by microbial spoilage or during in-tended processing of food of primary animal origin and their presence in-creases with maturation. Furthermore various drugs and others can inhibit histamine degradation or ac-tivate histamine release additionally.

Excessive supply of histamine 1) has to be reduced by a (hist)amine-poor diet and 2) can be reduced additionally by drugs, nutrients and supplements.

Pizza and red wine are taboo.

Helicobacter pylori infection as an environmental risk factor for migraine without aura

Yiannopoulou KG, Efthymiou A, Karydakis K, Arhimandritis A, Bovaretos N, Tzivras M

J Headache Pain. 2007; 8(6):329-33

Helicobacter pylori (H. pylori) infection has recently been associated with various extraintestinal pathologies and migraine. The aim of this study was to investigate the correlation of the H. pylori infection with the pathogenesis of migraine without aura, especially in cases not affected by endogenous risk factors, like hereditary pattern or hormonal fluctuations.A total of 49 outpatients (37 females and 12 males; age range: 19-47 years; mean age: 31,+/-14 years) affected by migraine without aura was evaluated. We divided them in 2 subgroups: a) with positive familial history, and/or with menstrual type of migraine b) with negative familial history and with menstrual unrelated type of migraine. H. pylori infection was diagnosed by the 13 C- urea breath test (INFAI - test). Control subjects consisted of 51 patients without any primary headache history (38 females; mean age of 32,+/-14,4 years; range 21-49 years), who underwent upper gastrointestinal (GI) endoscopy for investigation of anaemia or non ulcer dyspepsia. H. pylori detection was based on the histologic analysis of gastric mucosa biopsy. The prevalence of H. pylori infection was significantly higher in the migraineurs without aura compared to controls (p=0.016). The prevalence of H. pylori infection was significantly high in the mixed and in the female group of our patients without other predisposing factors for migraine without aura (81 and 87% respectively), while in the same groups with predisposing factors (menstruation and/or family history) the prevalence was only 36 and 37% respectively (p=0,001 for the first group and p=0,002 for the second group). Our results seem to highlight the role of H. pylori infection as a probable independent environmental risk factor for migraine without aura, especially in patients that are not genetically or hormonally susceptible to migraine.

[Histamine intolerance: the perils of biogenic amines] [Article in German]

Weiss J.

Am J Clin Nutr. 2007 May; 85(5):1185-96

2006

Eosinophilic esophagitis

Antón Remírez J, Escudero R, Cáceres O, Fernández-Benítez M.

Allergol Immunopathol (Madr). 2006 Mar-Apr; 34(2):79-81

BACKGROUND: Esophagitis is an increasingly diagnosed disease. Patients with gastroesophagic reflux, dysphagia, vomiting or abdominal pain, with a torpid response to the treatment, could be suffering from it.
MATERIAL AND METHODS: A 37 year-old male patient with background of gastroesophagic reflux and dysphagia for solids since 2002, self-limited diarrhea episodes and intolerance to alcoholic drinks due to epigastric pain. Skin prick tests, specific IgE, histamine release test and basophil activation test were carried out.
RESULTS: Skin prick test to the usual allergens with negative result; prick-prick tests to egg white and yolk, milk and apple with positive result to egg white; total serum IgE within normal levels, specific IgE to egg white with positive result; histamine release test (HRT) and basophil activation test (BAT) with positive result to egg white and yolk.
CONCLUSION: The patient was diagnosed eosinophilic esophagitis. The commercial food extracts have a great variability in their allergenic composition, which could result in false negative results in the prick test. Prick-prick with the natural food is a more sensitive technique than prick in the diagnosis of food allergy. There are other useful in vitro techniques, apart from specific IgE, in the diagnosis of food allergy. In our case, an exclusion diet of the involved food was more effective than other treatments for remission of the symptoms.

Histamine modulates mast cell degranulation through an indirect mechanism in a model IgE-mediated reaction

Carlos D, Sá-Nunes A, de Paula L, Matias-Peres C, Jamur MC, Oliver C, Serra MF, Martins MA, Faccioli LH

Eur J Immunol. 2006; 36(6): 1494-503

Histamine is released in inflammatory reactions and exerts an immunoregulatory function on cells present in the microenvironment. In this study, we compared the effect of histamine on degranulation of mast cells derived from animals bearing a parasitic infection with those from uninfected animals. Peritoneal mast cells (PMC) were obtained 24 days after infection of Wistar rats with Toxocara canis. The degree of degranulation was assessed either morphologically or by measuring the release of beta-hexosaminidase and TNF-alpha. Non-purified PMC or mast cells immunomagnetically purified with mAb AA4 were used. An increase in degranulation of non-purified mast cells from infected animals was observed after incubation with histamine in vitro or when histamine was injected into the peritoneal cavity. When a purified mast cell population was used, this effect was no longer observed. Supernatants from spleen cells stimulated with histamine induced degranulation of purified mast cells, and again, this was potentiated with PMC from infected animals. However, when supernatants from peritoneal macrophages similarly stimulated were used, a reduction in the degranulation of PMC from infected animals was observed. Our results suggest that histamine may act as a regulator of mast cell degranulation, thus modulating inflammatory responses due to infection with certain parasites.

Effect of sodium sulfite on mast cell degranulation and oxidant stress

Collaco CR, Hochman DJ, Goldblum RM, Brooks EG

Ann Allergy Asthma Immunol. 2006 Apr;96(4):550-6

BACKGROUND: Sulfur dioxide is 1 of 6 environmental pollutants monitored by the Environmental Protection Agency. Its ability to induce bronchoconstriction is well documented. It is highly soluble, initially forming sulfite ions in solution. Sulfur oxides are important constituents of other pollutants, such as diesel exhaust and fine particulates.
OBJECTIVE: To investigate the cellular responses of sulfite on cultured mast cells (rat basophilic leukemia [RBL-2H3] cells) and human peripheral blood basophils.
METHODS: Sulfite-induced mast cell degranulation and intracellular production of reactive oxygen species were evaluated in the presence and absence of antioxidants and inhibitors of redox metabolism. Degranulation was determined using beta-hexosaminidase, serotonin, and histamine release assays. Induction of intracellular reactive oxygen species generation was determined using the redox-sensitive dye 2',7'-dichlorofluorescein diacetate.
RESULTS: Sodium sulfite induced degranulation and the generation of intracellular reactive oxygen species in RBL-2H3 cells. These responses were inhibited by the free radical scavenger tetramethylthiourea and the flavoenzyme inhibitor diphenyliodinium but not by depletion of extracellular calcium. Peripheral blood basophils also showed histamine release after exposure to sodium sulfite
CONCLUSIONS: Sulfite, the aqueous ion of sulfur dioxide, induces cellular activation, leading to degranulation in mast cells through a non-IgE-dependent pathway. The response also differs from IgE-mediated degranulation in that it is insensitive to the influx of extracellular calcium. The putative pathway seems to rely on activation of the reduced form of nicotinamide adenine dinucleotide phosphate oxidase complex, leading to intracellular oxidative stress.

Severity of ulcerative colitis is associated with a polymorphism at diamine oxidase gene but not at histamine N-methyltransferase gene

García-Martin E, Mendoza JL, Martínez C, Taxonera C, Urcelay E, Ladero JM, de la Concha EG, Díaz-Rubio M, Agúndez JA.
World J Gastroenterol. 2006 ;12(4): 615-20
AIM: To analyse the role of two common polymorphisms in genes coding for histamine metabolising enzymes as it relates to the risk to develop ulcerative colitis (UC) and the clinical course of these patients.
METHODS: A cohort of 229 unrelated patients with UC recruited from a single centre and 261 healthy volunteers were analysed for the presence of Thr105Ile and His645Asp amino acid substitutions at histamine N-methyltransferase (HNMT) and diamine oxidase (ABP1) enzymes, respectively, by amplification-restriction procedures. All patients were phenotyped and followed up for at least 2 years (mean time 11 years).
RESULTS: There were no significant differences in the distribution of ABP1 alleles between ulcerative colitis patients and healthy individuals [OR (95% CI) for variant alleles=1.22 (0.91-1.61)]. However, mutated ABP1 alleles were present with higher frequency among the 58 patients that required immunosuppressive drugs [OR (95 % CI) for carriers of mutated alleles 2.41 (1.21-4.83; P=0.006)], with a significant gene-dose effect (P=0.0038). In agreement with the predominant role of ABP1 versus HNMT on local histamine metabolism in human bowel, the frequencies for carriers of HNMT genotypes or mutated alleles were similar among patients, regardless clinical evolution, and control individuals.
CONCLUSION: The His645Asp polymorphism of the histamine metabolising enzyme ABP1 is related to severity of ulcerative colitis.

Evidence for a reduced histamine degradation capacity in a subgroup of patients with atopic eczema

Maintz L, Benfadal S, Allam JP, Hagemann T, Fimmers R, Novak N.
J Allergy Clin Immunol. 2006 May; 117(5):1106-12
BACKGROUND: A diminished histamine degradation based on a reduced diaminoxidase activity is suspected as a reason for non-IgE-mediated food intolerance caused by histamine. Atopic eczema (AE) is often complicated by relapses triggered by IgE-mediated allergy to different kinds of food. However, in a subgroup of patients with AE, allergy testing proves negative, although these patients report a coherence of food intake and worsening of AE and describe symptoms that are very similar to histamine intolerance (HIT).
OBJECTIVES: It was the aim of our study to evaluate symptoms of HIT in combination with diaminoxidase levels in a total of 360 individuals consisting of patients with AE (n = 162) in comparison with patients with HIT (n = 124) without AE and healthy control volunteers (n = 85).
METHODS: Histamine plasma level was determined with an ELISA and diaminoxidase serum activity with the help of radio extraction assays using [3H]-labeled putrescine-dihydrochloride as a substrate. Detailed clinical evaluations of characteristic features of AE and HIT were performed.
RESULTS: Reduced diaminoxidase serum levels leading to occurrence of HIT symptoms like chronic headache, dysmenorrhea, flushing, gastrointestinal symptoms, and intolerance of histamine-rich food and alcohol were significantly more common in patients with AE than in controls. Reduction of both symptoms of HIT and Severity Scoring of Atopic Dermatitis could be achieved by a histamine-free diet in the subgroup of patients with AE and low diaminoxidase serum levels.
CONCLUSION: Higher histamine plasma levels combined with a reduced histamine degradation capacity might influence the clinical course of a subgroup of patients with AE.
CLINICAL IMPLICATIONS: As HIT emerges in a subgroup of patients with AE, a detailed anamnestic evaluation of food intolerance and HIT symptoms complemented by an allergological screening for food allergy, a diet diary, and, in confirmed suspicion of HIT, measurement of diaminoxidase activity and a histamine-free diet should be undertaken.

Food allergies and food intolerances

Ortolani C, Pastorello EA
Best Pract Res Clin Gastroenterol. 2006; 20(3):467-83
Adverse reactions to foods, aside from those considered toxic, are caused by a particular individual intolerance towards commonly tolerated foods. Intolerance derived from an immunological mechanism is referred to as Food Allergy, the non-immunological form is called Food Intolerance. IgE-mediated food allergy is the most common and dangerous type of adverse food reaction. It is initiated by an impairment of normal Oral Tolerance to food in predisposed individuals (atopic). Food allergy produces respiratory, gastrointestinal, cutaneous and cardiovascular symptoms but often generalized, life-threatening symptoms manifest at a rapid rate-anaphylactic shock. Diagnosis is made using medical history and cutaneous and serological tests but to obtain final confirmation a Double Blind Controlled Food Challenge must be performed. Food intolerances are principally caused by enzymatic defects in the digestive system, as is the case with lactose intolerance, but may also result from pharmacological effects of vasoactive amines present in foods (e.g. Histamine). Prevention and treatment are based on the avoidance of the culprit food.

Normobaric hypoxia and nitroglycerin as trigger factors for migraine

Schoonman GG, Sándor PS, Agosti RM, Siccoli M, Bärtsch P, Ferrari MD, Baumgartner RW
Cephalalgia. 2006; 26(7): 816-9
Migraine prevalence is increased in high-altitude populations and symptoms of acute mountain sickness mimic migraine symptoms. Here we tested whether normobaric hypoxia may trigger migraine attacks. As positive control we used nitrolgycerin (NTG), which has been shown to induce migraine attacks in up to 80% of migraineurs. Sixteen patients (12 females, mean age 28.9 +/- 7.2 years) suffering from migraine with (n = 8) and without aura (n = 8) underwent three different provocations (normobaric hypoxia, NTG and placebo) in a randomized, cross-over, double dummy design. Each provocation was performed on a separate day. The primary outcome measure was the proportion of patients developing a migraine attack according to the criteria of the International Headache Society within 8 h after provocation onset. Fourteen patients completed all three provocations. Migraine was provoked in six (42%) patients by hypoxia, in three (21%) by NTG and in two (14%) by placebo. The differences among groups were not significant (P = 0.197). The median time to attacks was 5 h. In conclusion, the (remarkably) low response rate to NTG is surprising in view of previous data. Further studies are required to establish fully the potency of hypoxia in triggering migraine attacks.
https://openaccess.leidenuniv.nl/bitstream/handle/1887/13094/5%20Ch3.pdf?sequence=5

2005

Structural basis for inhibition of histamine N-methyltransferase by diverse drugs
Horton JR, Sawada K, Nishibori M, Cheng X.
J Mol Biol. 2005 Oct 21;353(2):334-44
In mammals, histamine action is terminated through metabolic inactivation by histamine N-methyltransferase (HNMT) and diamine oxidase. In addition to three well-studied pharmacological functions, smooth muscle contraction, increased vascular permeability, and stimulation of gastric acid secretion, histamine plays important roles in neurotransmission, immunomodulation, and regulation of cell proliferation. The histamine receptor H1 antagonist diphenhydramine, the antimalarial drug amodiaquine, the antifolate drug metoprine, and the anticholinesterase drug tacrine (an early drug for Alzheimer's disease) are surprisingly all potent HNMT inhibitors, having inhibition constants in the range of 10-100nM. We have determined the structural mode of interaction of these four inhibitors with HNMT. Despite their structural diversity, they all occupy the histamine-binding site, thus blocking access to the enzyme's active site. Near the N terminus of HNMT, several aromatic residues (Phe9, Tyr15, and Phe19) adopt different rotamer conformations or become disordered in the enzyme-inhibitor complexes, accommodating the diverse, rigid hydrophobic groups of the inhibitors. The maximized shape complementarity between the protein aromatic side-chains and aromatic ring(s) of the inhibitors are responsible for the tight binding of these varied inhibitors.

Histamin-Intoleranz: Ein oft übersehenes Problem
Jarisch, R.
Arzt & Praxis 2005, 59 Jahrgang, Heft Nr. 908, 380-382

[Alimentary trigger factors that provoke migraine and tension-type headache.]
[Article in German]
Holzhammer J, Wober C.
Schmerz. 2005 Apr 2
Based on a review of the literature the authors discuss the role of nutrition in the precipitation of migraine and tension-type headache (TTH). The available information relies largely on the subjective assessment of the patients. Controlled trials suggest that alcohol and caffeine withdrawal are the most important nutritional precipitating factors of migraine and TTH. In addition, there is some evidence that missing meals is also an important factor. Dehydration seems to deserve more attention. A selective sensitivity to red wine has been shown in some patients, the importance of chocolate has been doubted seriously, and scientific evidence for cheese as a precipitating factor is lacking. Despite a series of experimental studies demonstrating that NO donors such as nitroglycerin and parenteral histamine cause headache the role of histamine, nitrates, and nitrites in food remains unclear. Similarly, other biogenic amines and aspartame have not been proven to precipitate headache. Sodium glutamate causes adverse reactions including headache probably at large doses ingested on an empty stomach. Therefore, patients should be advised that food plays a limited role as a precipitating factor of migraine and TTH. Subjective sensitivity to certain foods should be examined critically, and proven precipitating factors should be avoided. General dietary restrictions have not been proven to be useful.

Lack of association of histamine-N-methyltransferase (HNMT) polymorphisms with asthma in the Indian population
Sharma S, Mann D, Singh TP, Ghosh B
J Hum Genet. 2005; 50(12):611-7

Histamine plays a major role in allergic disorders, including asthma. A major pathway of histamine biotransformation in the lungs is mediated by histamine N-methyltransferase (HNMT). We investigated the association of a functional SNP C314T; a SNP A929G, a (CA)n repeat in intron 5, and a novel (CA)n repeat (BV677277), 7.5 kb downstream of the HNMT gene with asthma and its associated traits such as total serum IgE levels in a case-control as well as in a family-based study design. In contrast to a previous study, no association was observed for the polymorphisms investigated with asthma (P>0.05). When haplotypes were constructed for these loci and compared, no significant difference was observed in the distribution between cases and controls. In the family-based design, no biased transmission was observed for any of the polymorphisms and haplotypes with asthma using the additive model of inheritance in family-based association test (FBAT). Thus, consistent with the case-control findings, the polymorphisms and haplotypes in the HNMT gene are not associated with asthma in the Indian population.

Histamin und Kopfschmerz
Steinbrecher I, Jarisch R.
Allergologie 2005; 28: 84–91

Can Histamine in Wine Cause Adverse Reactions for Consumers?
Stockley C
2004 Annual Technical Issue of the Autralian & New Zealand Grapegrower & Windmaker, p. 77-82

Mastocytosis and adverse reactions to biogenic amines and histamine-releasing foods: what is the evidence?
Vlieg-Boerstra BJ, Heide S van der, Oude Elberink JNG, Kluin-Nelemans JC, Dubois AEJ
Netherlands J Med 2005; 63: 7
BACKGROUND: It has been suggested that normal concentrations of biogenic amines and 'histamine-releasing foods' may exacerbate symptoms in mastocytosis. The purpose of this study was to look for scientific evidence in the literature on diets restricted in biogenic amines and histamine-releasing foods in the treatment of mastocytosis.
METHODS: Medline (1966 to 2004), Cinahl (1982 to 2004) and the Cochraine Library were searched for double-blind placebo-controlled food challenge (DBPCFC) studies with biogenic amines and/or histamine-releasing foods in mastocytosis.
RESULTS: No studies employing DBPCFC with dietary biogenic amines or histamine-releasing foods in mastocytosis were found. Only a few in vitro studies in other diseases, animal studies and studies in humans in which histamine-releasing agents were incubated directly with duodenal tissues were found. One case was reported of severe adverse reactions to alcohol in mastocytosis, objectified by an open challenge.
CONCLUSION: Despite the widespread belief that biogenic amines and histamine-releasing foods may cause allergy-like, non-IgE-mediated symptoms in certain patients, the role of diets restricted in biogenic amines and histamine-releasing foods in the treatment of mastosytosis remains hypothetical but worthy of further investigation. There is some evidence for adverse reactions to alcohol in mastocytosis.

2004

Pseudoallergic reactions in chronic urticaria are associated with altered gastroduodenal permeability
Buhner S, Reese I, Kuehl F, Lochs H, Zuberbier T
Allergy 2004; 59: 1118–1123
BACKGROUND: In a subgroup of patients with chronic urticaria (CU) the disease is caused by pseudoallergic reactions to food. The aim of this study was to investigate whether disturbances of the gastrointestinal barrier function play a role in the pathomechanism of the disease.
METHODS: In 55 patients with CU gastrointestinal permeability was measured with an in vivo triple-sugar-test before and after 24 days of a diet low in pseudoallergens. Sucrose served as marker for gastroduodenal permeability, lactulose/mannitol ratio for intestinal permeability.
RESULTS: Basal gastroduodenal and intestinal permeability were significantly higher in patients with urticaria as compared to controls. In 29 of the 55 patients skin symptoms decreased or completely disappeared during the diet (respond-ers). Compared to nonresponders (n¼26), responders had a significantly higher gastroduodenal permeability before treatment (0.36 ± 0.04 vs $0.15 \pm 0.01\%$ sucrose; $P< 0.001$), which decreased after the diet (0.17 ± 0.02; $P< 0.001$).
The number of patients with Helicobacter pylori infections did not differ between the two groups.
CONCLUSIONS: The results indicate that in a subgroup of patients with CU and pseudoallergy an impaired gastroduodenal barrier function may be of patho-physiological importance. The underlying mechanisms seem to be independent of H. pyloriinfection.

Overview of the role of alcohol dehydrogenase and aldehyde dehydrogenase and their variants in the genesis of alcohol-related pathology

Crabb DW, Matsumoto M, Chang D, You M
Proc Nutr Soc. 2004;63(1): 49-63

Histamin-Intoleranz. Histamin und Seekrankheit
R. Jarisch
ISBN 3-13-105382-8, Publisher Georg Thieme Verlag, Stuttgart

Review: Mast cells in inflammatory arthritis
Nigrovic PA, Lee DM
Arthritis Res Ther 2005, 7:1-11

Mast cells are present in limited numbers in normal human synovium, but in rheumatoid arthritis and other inflammatory joint diseases this population can expand to constitute 5% or more of all synovial cells. Recent investigations in a murine model have demonstrated that mast cells can have a critical role in the generation of inflammation within the joint. This finding highlights the results of more than 20 years of research indicating that mast cells are frequent participants in non-allergic immune responses as well as in allergy. Equipped with a diversity of surface receptors and effector capabilities, mast cells are sentinels of the immune system, detecting and delivering a first response to invading bacteria and other insults. Accumulating within inflamed tissues, mast cells produce cytokines and other mediators that may contribute vitally to ongoing inflammation. Here we review some of the non-allergic functions of mast cells and focus on the potential role of these cells in murine and human inflammatory arthritis.

Histamine intolerance-like symptoms in healthy volunteers after oral provocation with liquid histamine
Wöhrl S, Hemmer W, Focke M, Rappersberger K, Jarisch R.
Allergy Asthma Proc. 2004 Sep-Oct; 25(5):305-11

Histamine in food at non-toxic doses has been proposed to be a major cause of food intolerance causing symptoms like diarrhea, hypotension, headache, pruritus and flush ("histamine intolerance"). Histamine-rich foods such as cheese, sausages, sauerkraut, tuna, tomatoes, and alcoholic beverages may contain histamine up to 500 mg/kg. We conducted a randomized, double-blind, placebo-controlled cross-over study in 10 healthy females (age range 22-36 years, mean 29.1 +/- 5.4) who were hospitalized and challenged on two consecutive days with placebo (peppermint tea) or 75 mg of pure histamine (equaling 124 mg histamine dihydrochloride, dissolved in peppermint tea). Objective parameters (heart rate, blood pressure, skin temperature, peak flow) as well as a total clinical symptom score using a standardized protocol were recorded at baseline, 10, 20, 40, 80 minutes, and 24 hours. The subjects received a histamine-free diet also low in allergen 24 hours before hospitalization and over the whole observation period. Blood samples were drawn at baseline, 10, 20, 40, and 80 minutes, and histamine and the histamine-degrading enzyme diamine oxidase (DAO) were determined. After histamine challenge, 5 of 10 subjects showed no reaction. One individual experienced tachycardia, mild hypotension after 20 minutes, sneezing, itching of the nose, and rhinorrhea after 60 minutes. Four subjects experienced delayed symptoms like diarrhea (4x), flatulence (3x), headache (3x), pruritus (2x) and ocular symptoms (1x) starting 3 to 24 hours after provocation. No subject reacted to placebo. No changes were observed in histamine and DAO levels within the first 80 minutes in non-reactors as well as reactors. There was no difference in challenge with histamine versus challenge with placebo. We conclude that 75 mg of pure liquid oral histamine--a dose found in normal meals--can provoke immediate as well as delayed symptoms in 50% of healthy females without a history of food intolerance.

2003

[Immediate hypersensitivity is rarely implicated in drug induced urticaria] [Article in French]
Cousin F, Catelain A, Philips K, Favier B, Queuille E, Nicolas JF.
Ann Dermatol Venereol. 2003 Mar; 130(3):321-4

INTRODUCTION: The unexpected appearance of acute urticaria during the course of drug treatment gives rise to the following question: is it an allergic urticaria (due to an immediate hypersensitivity: IgE mediated specific immunity) or is it pseudo-allergic? We report our findings in an immuno-allergological study of patients who were sent for drug intolerance which presented as immediate hypersensivity (urticaria, angiooedema, anaphylactic shock).
METHODS: A prospective study was conducted including all the patients who were sent to the unit for urticaria or angiooedema type drug intolerance. Patients were questioned about previous chronic urticaria and also about urticaria after taking different medicines. The clinical examination looked for a dermographism. All the patients then took skin tests for immediate hypersensitivity, the molecule was contra-indicated and tests for cross-reactivity were conducted.
PATIENTS: Three hundred fifty patients were sent to this unit between February 2000 and April 2001 for drug intolerance, mostly with urticaria/angiooedema but in 7 cases with anaphylactic shock. The

incriminated drugs were varied: 50 p. 100 were due mainly to penicillins and cephalosporins. Other drug groups were also involved: non steroid anti-inflammatories, aspirin and paracetamol for the most part, along with local anesthetics, morphine-based products, contrast iodine products, corticosteroids. RESULTS: Of the 350 patients tested, only 22 were allergic and had positive tests for the incriminated drug. In these 22 patients, with the exception of 2 of them, the effects were severe (anaphylactic shock in 7 patients) and the urticaria was only a minor manifestation of the reaction. The drugs responsible were cephalosporin (10 patients), the penicillin (6 patients), insulin (2 patients), gonadorelin (1 patient), carboxymethylcellulose (1 patient), lidocain (1 patient), and sulfamethoxazole (1 patient). The 328 other patients had negative tests and were able to retake the tested molecule without incident. Most of them had antecedents of chronic urticaria or dermographism.
DISCUSSION: Only 22 patients of the 350, i.e. 6 p. 100 were genuinely allergic. These patients were those who presented the most severe symptoms. The other patients, i.e. the majority, suffered from pseudo-allergic drug-induced urticaria, which made retaking the medicines possible.

Histamine H4 receptor mediates chemotaxis and calcium mobilization of mast cells

Hofstra CL, Desai PJ, Thurmond RL, Fung-Leung WP
J Pharmacol Exp Ther. 2003; 305(3): 1212-21
The diverse physiological functions of histamine are mediated through distinct histamine receptors. Mast cells are major producers of histamine, yet effects of histamine on mast cells are currently unclear. The present study shows that histamine induces chemotaxis of mouse mast cells, without affecting mast cell degranulation. Mast cell chemotaxis toward histamine could be blocked by the dual H3/H4 receptor antagonist thioperamide, but not by H1 or H2 receptor antagonists. This chemotactic response is mediated by the H4 receptor, because chemotaxis toward histamine was absent in mast cells derived from H4 receptor-deficient mice but was detected in H3 receptor-deficient mast cells. In addition, Northern blot analysis showed the expression of H4 but not H3 receptors on mast cells. Activation of H4 receptors by histamine resulted in calcium mobilization from intracellular calcium stores. Both G alpha i/o proteins and phospholipase C (PLC) are involved in histamine-induced calcium mobilization and chemotaxis in mast cells, because these responses were completely inhibited by pertussis toxin and PLC inhibitor 1-[6-[[17 beta-3-methoxyestra-1,3,5 (10)-trien-17-yl]amino]hexyl]-1H-pyrrole-2,5-dione (U73122). In summary, histamine was shown to mediate signaling and chemotaxis of mast cells via the H4 receptor. This mechanism might be responsible for mast cell accumulation in allergic tissues.

Effect of Heat Treatment on Lipid Stability in Processed Oats

Lehtinen P., Kiiliäinen K, Lehtomäki I, and Laakso S
Journal of Cereal Science 37 (2003) 215-221
The shelf life of processed oat products and the usability of oats in modern food formulations are in many cases still limited by the lipid-associated deterioration. To elucidate the role of lipase inactivation in the development of rancidity in oats, heat treatments varying in severity were applied. Effects of these treatments on lipase activity and lipid oxidation were studied either directly after processing by mixing the fractions in water or after a long-term storage of dry fractions. A trend was found, that the lower the residual lipase activity in whole kernels or kernel fractions, the higher was the oxidation of lipids and evolution of volatile oxidation products during prolonged storage of the dry fractions. If bran was heat-treated to zero lipase activity, the amount of headspace hexanal detected after 12-month storage was 5 to 7 times larger than detected in non-heat treated bran. This formation of hexanal was linked to the oxidation of polar lipids. If the heat treatment was totally omitted, the oxidation of unsaturated fatty acids in polar lipids did not occur even during prolonged storage. The oxidation of polar lipids suggests heat-induced disintegration of membrane structures and inactivation of heat labile antioxidants. This study identifes heat treatments as critical control points in obtaining oat products with enhanced self-stability.

The diet factor in pediatric and adolescent migraine

Millichap JG, Yee MM
Pediatr Neurol. 2003; 28(1): 9-15
Diet can play an important role in the precipitation of headaches in children and adolescents with migraine. The diet factor in pediatric migraine is frequently neglected in favor of preventive drug therapy. The list of foods, beverages, and additives that trigger migraine includes cheese, chocolate, citrus fruits, hot dogs, monosodium glutamate, aspartame, fatty foods, ice cream, caffeine withdrawal, and alcoholic drinks, especially red wine and beer. Underage drinking is a significant potential cause of recurrent headache in today's adolescent patients. Tyramine, phenylethylamine, histamine, nitrites, and sulfites are involved in the mechanism of food intolerance headache. Immunoglobulin E-mediated food allergy is an infrequent cause. Dietary triggers affect phases of the migraine process by influencing release of serotonin and norepinephrine, causing vasoconstriction or vasodilatation, or by direct stimulation of trigeminal ganglia, brainstem, and cortical neuronal pathways. Treatment begins with a headache and diet diary and the selective avoidance of foods presumed to trigger attacks. A universal migraine diet with simultaneous elimination of all potential food triggers is generally not

advised in practice. A well-balanced diet is encouraged, with avoidance of fasting or skipped meals. Long-term prophylactic drug therapy is appropriate only after exclusion of headache-precipitating trigger factors, including dietary factors.

Intolerance to dietary biogenic amines: a review
Jansen SC, van Dusseldorp M, Bottema KC, Dubois AE.
Ann Allergy Asthma Immunol. 2003 Sep; 91(3):233-40; quiz 241-2, 296
OBJECTIVE: To evaluate the scientific evidence for purported intolerance to dietary biogenic amines.
DATA SOURCES: MEDLINE was searched for articles in the English language published between January 1966 and August 2001. The keyword biogenic amin* was combined with hypersens*, allerg*, intoler*, and adverse. Additionally, the keywords histamine, tyramine, and phenylethylamine were combined with headache, migraine, urticaria, oral challenge, and oral provocation. Articles were also selected from references in relevant literature.
STUDY SELECTION: Only oral challenge studies in susceptible patients were considered. Studies with positive results (ie, studies in which an effect was reported) were only eligible when a randomized, double-blind, placebo-controlled design was used. Eligible positive result studies were further evaluated according to a number of scientific criteria. Studies with negative results (ie, studies in which no effect was reported) were examined for factors in their design or methods that could be responsible for a false-negative outcome. Results of methodologically weak or flawed studies were considered inconclusive.
RESULTS: A total of 13 oral challenge studies (5 with positive results and 8 with negative results) were found. Three of them (all with positive results) were considered ineligible. By further evaluation of the 10 eligible studies, 6 were considered inconclusive. The 4 conclusive studies all reported negative results. One conclusive study showed no relation between biogenic amines in red wine and wine intolerance. Two conclusive studies found no effect of tyramine on migraine. One conclusive study demonstrated no relation between the amount of phenylethylamine in chocolate and headache attacks in individuals with headache.
CONCLUSIONS: The current scientific literature shows no relation between the oral ingestion of biogenic amines and food intolerance reactions. There is therefore no scientific basis for dietary recommendations concerning biogenic amines in such patients.

Blood levels of homocysteine, folate, vitamin B6 and B12 in women using oral contraceptives compared to non-users.
Lussana F, Zighetti ML, Bucciarelli P, Cugno M, Cattaneo M.
Thromb Res. 2003; 112(1-2): 37-41
BACKGROUND AND OBJECTIVES: To compare the levels of total homocysteine (tHcy), folate, vitamin B6 and B12, in women not using oral contraceptives (OC) vs. those using OC.
MATERIALS AND METHODS: 219 healthy women were enrolled in the study; 159 of them had not been using OC for at least 12 months prior to their enrollment, while 60 were on regular OC treatment.
RESULTS: The median levels of vitamin B6 and B12 were significantly lower in OC users than in non-users (24.2 vs. 32.9 nmol/l, p=0.029; 278 vs. 429 ng/ml, p<0.001). There were no statistically significant differences in the levels of tHcy (fasting and post-methionine loading) and folate.
CONCLUSIONS: In our cross-sectional study, OC use was associated with low vitamin B6 and B12 levels. Since low vitamin B6 levels are independently associated with heightened risks for arterial and venous thromboembolism (TE), they could partly account for the increased TE risk of OC users.

The diet factor in pediatric and adolescent migraine
Millichap JG, Yee MM.
Pediatr Neurol. 2003 Jan; 28(1):9-15
Diet can play an important role in the precipitation of headaches in children and adolescents with migraine. The diet factor in pediatric migraine is frequently neglected in favor of preventive drug therapy. The list of foods, beverages, and additives that trigger migraine includes cheese, chocolate, citrus fruits, hot dogs, monosodium glutamate, aspartame, fatty foods, ice cream, caffeine withdrawal, and alcoholic drinks, especially red wine and beer. Underage drinking is a significant potential cause of recurrent headache in today's adolescent patients. Tyramine, phenylethylamine, histamine, nitrites, and sulfites are involved in the mechanism of food intolerance headache. Immunoglobulin E-mediated food allergy is an infrequent cause. Dietary triggers affect phases of the migraine process by influencing release of serotonin and norepinephrine, causing vasoconstriction or vasodilatation, or by direct stimulation of trigeminal ganglia, brainstem, and cortical neuronal pathways. Treatment begins with a headache and diet diary and the selective avoidance of foods presumed to trigger attacks. A universal migraine diet with simultaneous elimination of all potential food triggers is generally not advised in practice. A well-balanced diet is encouraged, with avoidance of fasting or skipped meals. Long-term prophylactic drug therapy is appropriate only after exclusion of headache-precipitating trigger factors, including dietary factors.

[Allergic and pseudo-allergic reactions to foods in chronic urticaria][Article in French]
Moneret-Vautrin DA.

Ann Dermatol Venereol. 2003 May; 130 Spec No 1:1S35-42

The fact that more than 30 p. 100 of patients with chronic urticaria incriminate foods, and that acute urticaria is a frequent symptom of food allergy, argue in favour of a systematic search for food involvement in chronic urticaria. A global overview of publications through Medline selects 49 out of 189 papers upon strict criteria, devoted to the links between chronic urticaria and foods. Possible links exist between chronic urticaria and intolerance to additives, intolerance or allergy to contaminants, pseudo-allergic reactions to foods and IgE-dependent food allergy. The diagnosis of intolerance to additives relies on double blind placebo-controlled oral challenges, showing positivity in 2 to 3 p. 100 of cases. Flavours are being suspected but have not been validated by such oral challenges. Contaminants are nickel salts, penicillin residues in meats and milk, Anisakis larvae in fish. Intolerance to biogenic amines could be somewhat frequent and is well-documented by experimental studies of the metabolism of histamine and by the results of specific diets with a low content of amines. IgE-dependent food allergy has been evidenced in 1 to 5 p. 100 of cases. The author puts forward a methodology to search for the implication of foods in chronic urticaria, restricting the search to non-inflammatory CU, discarding moreover chronic urticaria due to physical agents, or to contact. Idiopathic chronic urticaria, that might include a subgroup of auto-immune chronic urticaria is under scope. A preliminary study of the regimen during one week needs to be carried out in order to detect an excess of consumption of categories of foods inducing pseudo-allergic reactions, or of additives. An eviction diet for biogenic amines may be proposed first. Its failure may lead to skin prick tests to foods that are daily consumed. Biological tests are not advised. When sensitization is confirmed, a 3 week eviction of the food comes ahead of a double blind placebo-controlled oral challenge. The positivity indicates that this food is likely to be a causal agent and the diagnosis can finally be based on the recovery after the implementation of strict avoidance diets.

Analysis of genetic polymorphisms of enzymes involved in histamine metabolism
Petersen J, Drasche A, Raithel M, Schwelberger HG

Inflamm Res. 2003 Apr;52 Suppl 1:S69-70

Evaluation of the effects of Neptune Krill Oil on the management of premenstrual syndrome and dysmenorrhea
Sampalis F, Bunea R, Pelland MF, Kowalski O, Duguet N, Dupuis S.

Altern Med Rev. 2003 May;8(2):171-9

PRIMARY OBJECTIVE: To evaluate the effectiveness of Neptune Krill Oil (NKO) for the management of premenstrual syndrome and dysmenorrhea.
SECONDARY OBJECTIVE: To compare the effectiveness of NKO for the management of premenstrual syndrome and dysmenorrhea with that of omega-3 fish oil. METHODS/ DESIGN: Double-blind, randomized clinical trial.
SETTING: Outpatient clinic.
PARTICIPANTS: Seventy patients of reproductive age diagnosed with premenstrual syndrome according to the Diagnostic and Statistical Manual of Mental Disorders, Third Edition, Revised (DSM-III-R).
INTERVENTIONS: Treatment period of three months with either NKO or omega-3 fish oil.
OUTCOME MEASURES: Self-Assessment Questionnaire based on the American College of Obstetricians and Gynecologists (ACOG) diagnostic criteria for premenstrual syndrome and dysmenorrhea and number of analgesics used for dysmenorrhea.
RESULTS: In 70 patients with complete data, a statistically significant improvement was demonstrated among baseline, interim, and final evaluations in the self assessment questionnaire ($P < 0.001$) within the NKO group as well as between-group comparison to fish oil, after three cycles or 45 and 90 days of treatment. Data analysis showed a significant reduction of the number of analgesics used for dysmenorrhea within the NKO group (comparing baseline vs. 45- vs. 90-day visit). The between-groups analysis illustrated that women taking NKO consumed significantly fewer analgesics during the 10-day treatment period than women receiving omega-3 fish oil ($P < 0.03$).
CONCLUSION: Neptune Krill Oil can significantly reduce dysmenorrhea and the emotional symptoms of premenstrual syndrome and is shown to be significantly more effective for the complete management of premenstrual symptoms compared to omega-3 fish oil.

Clinical significance of plasma diamine oxidase activity in pediatric patients: influence of nutritional therapy and chemotherapy
Tanaka Y, Mizote H, Asakawa T, Kobayashi H, Otani M, Tanikawa K, Nakamizo H, Kawaguchi C, Asagiri K, Akiyoshi K, Hikida S, Nakamura T.

Source: Kurume Med J. 2003;50(3-4):131-7

The aims of this study were to determine the normal values of plasma diamine oxidase (pDAO) activity in children and to examine the influence of several factors (nutritional management, dietary fiber, and chemotherapy) on pDAO activity. The activity of pDAO was measured in 138 healthy children with minor surgical conditions such as inguinal hernia or undescended testis. In order to define normal values patients were subdivided into 5 groups according to age. Next, changes in pDAO activity under different nutritional conditions were studied in 14 patients with adhesive ileus. The influence of chemotherapeutic drugs on pDAO activity was also studied in 19 neuroblastoma patients. I. The normal values of pDAO activity at year < 1, 1 < or = years < 3, 3 < or = years < 6.6 < or = years < 12, 12 < or = years were 6.65 +/- 1.75, 7.70 +/- 2.29, 6.53 +/- 1.68, 5.85 +/- 1.87, 5.06 +/- 1.84 units/l, respectively. II. The pDAO activities in patients with ileus were 4.73 +/- 1.02 (total parenteral nutrition), 6.84 +/- 1.18 (enteral, nutrition), 7.62 +/- 0.67 (soluble dietary fiber added enteral nutrition) and 8.82 +/- 1.26 units/l (oral feeding). The difference in pDAO activity at enteral or oral feeding vs. total parenteral nutrition was significant (p < .0001). III. The pDAO activity decreased significantly and remained low during the first 4 days after cyclophosphamide administration in neuroblastoma patients. The preadministration of dietary fiber inhibited the influence of cyclophosphamide. Plasma DAO activity was greatly influenced by nutritional management and administration of dietary fiber and/or cyclophosphamide. Plasma DAO activity may be a sensitive marker of intestinal function in children.

Histamine stimulates the proliferation of human articular chondrocytes in vitro and is expressed by chondrocytes in osteoarthritic cartilage
Tetlow LC, Woolley DE
Ann Rheum Dis 2003;62: 991-994
OBJECTIVES: To determine the effects of histamine on the proliferative rate of human articular chondrocytes (HAC) in vitro, and to demonstrate whether HAC in osteoarthritic (OA) cartilage express histamine and histidine decarboxylase (HDC).
METHODS: HAC in vitro were incubated with and without histamine in 96 well culture plates and the extent of cell proliferation was determined using the naphthol blue-black method. Histamine effects were analysed with the histamine H1 and H2 receptor antagonists, mepyramine and ranitidine, respectively. Rabbit polyclonal antibodies and alkaline phosphatase conjugated secondary antibodies were used, and histamine and HDC were demonstrated by immunohistochemistry in OA cartilage tissues.
RESULTS: Histamine stimulated the proliferation of HAC in culture. This stimulation was blocked by the addition of mepyramine, but not ranitidine, suggesting that the effect is mediated through H1 histamine receptors. The addition of α-fluoromethylhistidine, a specific inhibitor of histidine decarboxylase (the enzyme responsible for histamine production), reduced the rate of proliferation of HAC. Both histamine and histidine decarboxylase were demonstrated in chondrocytes of OA cartilage by immunohistochemistry.
CONCLUSIONS: Changes induced by histamine in the proliferative rate of HAC may contribute to the formation of chondrocyte clusters associated with OA cartilage; an observation supported by the demonstration of histamine and HDC expression by chondrocytes of OA cartilage in situ.

Allergic and asthmatic reactions to alcoholic drinks
Vally H, Thompson PJ
Addict Biol. 2003 Mar; 8(1):3-11
Alcoholic drinks are capable of triggering a wide range of allergic and allergic-like responses, including rhinitis, itching, facial swelling, headache, cough and asthma. Limited epidemiological data suggests that many individuals are affected and that sensitivities occur to a variety of drinks, including wine, beer and spirits. In surveys of asthmatics, over 40% reported the triggering of allergic or allergic-like symptoms following alcoholic drink consumption and 30 - 35% reported worsening of their asthma. Sensitivity to ethanol itself can play a role in triggering adverse responses, particularly in Asians, which is due mainly to a reduced capacity to metabolize acetaldehyde. In Caucasians, specific non-alcohol components are the main cause of sensitivities to alcoholic drinks. Allergic sensitivities to specific components of beer, spirits and distilled liquors have been described. Wine is clearly the most commonly reported trigger for adverse responses. Sensitivities to wine appear to be due mainly to pharmacological intolerances to specific components, such as biogenic amines and the sulphite additives. Histamine in wine has been associated with the triggering of a wide spectrum of adverse symptoms, including sneezing, rhinitis, itching, flushing, headache and asthma. The sulphite additives in wine have been associated with triggering asthmatic responses. Clinical studies have confirmed sensitivities to the sulphites in wine in limited numbers of individuals, but the extent to which the sulphites contribute to wine sensitivity overall is not clear. The aetiology of wine-induced asthmatic responses may be complex and may involve several co-factors.

2002

Use of gas chromatography-olfactometry to identify key odorant compounds in dark chocolate. Comparison of samples before and after conching
Counet C, Callemien D, Ouwerx C, Collin S
J Agric Food Chem. 2002; 50(8): 2385-91

After vacuum distillation and liquid-liquid extraction, the volatile fractions of dark chocolates were analyzed by gas chromatography-olfactometry and gas chromatography-mass spectrometry. Aroma extract dilution analysis revealed the presence of 33 potent odorants in the neutral/basic fraction. Three of these had a strong chocolate flavor: 2-methylpropanal, 2-methylbutanal, and 3-methylbutanal. Many others were characterized by cocoa/praline-flavored/nutty/coffee notes: 2,3-dimethylpyrazine, trimethylpyrazine, tetramethylpyrazine, 3(or 2),5-dimethyl-2(or 3)-ethylpyrazine, 3,5(or 6)-diethyl-2-methylpyrazine, and furfurylpyrrole. Comparisons carried out before and after conching indicate that although no new key odorant is synthesized during the heating process, levels of 2-phenyl-5-methyl-2-hexenal, Furaneol, and branched pyrazines are significantly increased while most Strecker aldehydes are lost by evaporation.

Idiopathic anaphylaxis
Ring J, Darsow U.
Curr Allergy Asthma Rep. 2002 Jan; 2(1):40-5
Anaphylaxis represents the maximal variant of an immediate-type allergic reaction involving the whole organism with manifestations in different organ systems. IgE-mediated mast cell and basophil activation is the major pathomechanism; however, immune complex and pseudo-allergic reactions also may lead to the same symptomatology. The most common elicitors are drugs, additives, occupational substances, animal venoms, aeroallergens, and contact urticariogens but also physical factors (cold, heat, ultraviolet light, exercise). When no eliciting factors can be detected, the term "idiopathic anaphylaxis" is used. The diagnosis of idiopathic anaphylaxis is, therefore, a diagnosis of exclusion and may be made only after careful allergy history taking and diagnosis involving in vitro tests. Possible mechanisms underlying the pathophysiology of idiopathic anaphylaxis include undetected diseases (eg, mastocytosis occulta), concomitant anaphylaxis-enhancing medication (b-blockers), secretion of histamine-releasing factor from T lymphocytes, autoantibodies against IgE or IgE receptors, and angiotensin II deficiency. One of the many differential diagnoses of anaphylaxis may have been overlooked. The treatment of idiopathic anaphylaxis follows the rules of antianaphylactic therapy.

[Histamine receptors in the female reproductive system. Part I. Role of the mast cells and histamine in female reproductive system].[Article in Polish]
Szelag A, Merwid-Lad A, Trocha M.
Ginekol Pol. 2002 Jul;73(7):627-35
Histamine isolated from many different tissues, acts via three types of histamine receptors: H1, H2 and H3. In peripheral tissues histamine is mainly stored in mast cells (MC). Presence of mast cells was proved also in mammals' uteri. In human uterus the majority of mast cells are located close to smooth muscle cells. It might indicate that MC plays a role in tissue remodelling during the menstrual cycle. The quantity and activity of mast cells is in connection with hormonal status of the organism. Although there are some differences, human uterine mast cells are similar to the mast cells isolated from other tissues. It is suggested that histamine is important for normal ovulation, blastocyst implantation, placental blood flow regulation, lactation and contractile activity of uterus. Histamine may also play a role in pathological processes such as pre-eclampsia or preterm delivery. The participation of mast cells and histamine in blastocyst implantation is very controversial. In W/Wv mice (without mast cells) normal implantation was observed. It denies the main role of mast cells in this process but dos not exclude histamine action. In mice the major source of histamine are uterine epithelial cells during early pregnancy. The influence of cytokines on blastocyst implantation and the role of histamine in cytokines release from the uterine mast cells are also very unclear.

[Histamine receptors in the female reproductive system. Part II. The role of histamine in the placenta, histamine receptors and the uterus contractility] [Article in Polish]
Szelag A, Merwid-Lad A, Trocha M.
Ginekol Pol. 2002 Jul;73(7):636-44
The presence of the mast cells was confirmed not only in the uterus but also in the placental tissue. Mediators released from the placental mast cells may play a role in regulation of placental blood flow and normal blood pressure. Processes such uptake and clearance of vasoactive mediators may be upset in those women who developed pre-eclampsia. Histamine released from the placental mast cells may be involved in the mechanisms controlling myometrium contractility during the labour at term and preterm delivery. There is a correlation between the level of placental histamine and presence (or not) uterus contractility. Histamine produce a contractile response in isolated myometrial strips, in the majority of mammals, via H1 histamine receptors activation, but in some species e.g. rat, predominant response of uterus is relaxation (via H2 histamine receptors activation). Predominant response of the human uterus to histamine is contraction. Relaxation of human myometrial strips may be evoked after earlier usage of H1 receptors antagonists, although some H2 receptors agonists (e.g. dimaprit) induce the relaxation of human uterus without H1 receptors antagonists. Myometrium contractile activity is under control of sexual hormones. Neither the presence of H3 histamine receptors on the human myometrial smooth cells nor its role in the female reproductive system

regulation was proved. Lack of the functional H3 receptors either on the smooth muscle cells or neuronal components of the animals' myometrium was shown in some studies.

[Revised terminology for allergies and related conditions] [Article in Dutch]
van Wijk G.R, van Cauwenberge PB, Johansson SG.
Ned Tijdschr Geneeskd. 2002 Nov 30; 146(48):2289-93
The European Academy of Allergology and Clinical Immunology has proposed a revised terminology for allergic and allergy-related reactions that can be used independently of target organ or patient age group. The proposed terminology is based on the present knowledge of the mechanisms which initiate and mediate allergic reactions. 'Hypersensitivity' is an umbrella term, 'allergy' involves a hypersensitivity reaction which is initiated by an immunological mechanism, and 'atopy' is an individual or familial tendency to produce IgE antibodies in response to low doses of allergens, and is accompanied by the typical symptoms or asthma rhino-conjunctivitis or eczema/dermatitis. Each condition should be categorised as 'allergic/not allergic', and the allergic conditions should be further categorised as 'IgE-mediated/non IgE-mediated' (sometimes: 'IgE-associated'). Terms which are no longer in use include: 'idiosyncrasy' (this will now become 'hypersensitivity'); 'pseudo-allergy' ('non-allergic hypersensitivity'); 'extrinsic', 'intrinsic', 'endogenous' and 'exogenous asthma' ('allergic' (possibly 'IgE-mediated') and 'non-allergic asthma'); 'atopic eczema' ('atopic eczema/dermatitis syndrome': 'allergic (possibly 'IgE-mediated') or 'non-allergic'); 'intrinsic' and 'cryptogenic variants of eczema' ('non-allergic atopic eczema/dermatitis syndrome'); 'food intolerance' ('non-allergic food hypersensitivity') and 'anaphylactoid reaction' ('non-allergic anaphylaxis').

Aromatic components of food as novel eliciting factors of pseudoallergic reactions in chronic urticaria
Zuberbier T, Pfrommer C, Specht K, Vieths S, Bastl-Borrmann R, Worm M, Henz BM.
J Allergy Clin Immunol. 2002 Feb;109(2):343-8
BACKGROUND: Pseudoallergic reactions (PARs) against both additives and natural foods have been reported to elicit chronic urticaria, but in natural food the responsible ingredients are largely unknown.
OBJECTIVE: The study was aimed at identifying novel pseudoallergens in food and focused on evaluating tomatoes, white wine, and herbs as frequently reported food items eliciting wheal responses in urticaria.
METHODS: In 33 patients with chronic urticaria and PARs to food (proved by means of elimination diet and subsequent re-exposure with provocation meals), oral provocation tests were performed with field-grown tomatoes, organically grown white wine (whole food, steam distillates, and residues), oily extracts from herbs, and food additives. In addition, skin biopsy specimens from patients were studied for in vitro mast-cell histamine release with tomato distillate alone or on subsequent stimulation with anti-IgE, substance P, and C5a.
RESULTS: Seventy-six percent of patients reacted to whole tomato (steam distillate, 45%; residue, 15%), 50% to food additives, 47% to herbs, and 44% to whole wine (extract, 27%; residue, 0%). Histamine, protein, and high levels of salicylate were only found in residues. The tomato distillate was further analyzed by means of mass spectroscopy, identifying low molecular-weight aldehydes, ketones, and alcohol as major ingredients. In vitro histamine release was not caused by tomato extract itself but was enhanced by means of subsequent stimulation with substance P and C5a but not by anti-IgE.
CONCLUSION: Aromatic volatile ingredients in food are novel agents eliciting PARs in chronic urticaria. Histamine, salicylate, and a direct mast-cell histamine release are not involved in this reactivity to naturally occurring pseudoallergens.

2001

[The hypo-allergic diet][Article in German]
Ballmer-Weber BK.
Ther Umsch. 2000 Mar; 57(3):121-7
A hypoallergenic diet in a proper sense does not exist. The prescription of a dietary treatment for allergic diseases or intolerance reactions is highly dependent on an exact allergologic diagnosis. An IgE-mediated allergy to food is treated by an elimination diet. In chronic disease, e.g. chronic urticaria or chronic abdominal symptoms, the relevance of specific IgE to food allergens can be proved by a diagnostic elimination diet, which is followed by oral provocation. In children at risk for atopic diseases (one or both parents or siblings with atopic diseases) a preventive diet during the first year of life is recommended. The cornerstones of such a diet are breast feeding during the first six months of life, late introduction of solid food and the avoidance of allergenic proteins such as cow's milk, eggs and fish during the first year of life. In intolerance reaction an additive free diet or a diet with low content of biogenic amines may be recommended. Patients with chronic urticaria or atopic dermatitis may suffer from an intolerance to histamine. A diet with a low content of biogenic amines may improve the condition of these patients.

[Pseudoallergies][Article in Italian]

Bernardini R, Novembre E, Lombardi E, Monaco MG, Monte MT, Pucci N, Rossi ME, Vierucci A.
Pediatr Med Chir. 2001 Jan-Feb; 23(1):9-16
Pseudo-allergic-reactions (PAR) are clinical manifestations including urticaria, angioedema, conjunctivitis, rhinitis, asthma, and anaphylaxis. The prevalence of PAR ranges from 0.1% to 75% according to various studies. The pathogenetic mechanism of these diseases is not immunologically mediated. Food, additives, and drugs are the main responsibilities for PAR. The diagnosis of PAR is characterized by the absence of specific IgE for the suspected products. The absence of immunological mechanisms is confirmed by in vitro and in vivo tests. The treatment of PAR is similar to that of allergic diseases (antihistamine drugs, steroids, B2 agonists, epinephrine).

Constitutive hyperhistaminaemia: a possible mechanism for recurrent anaphylaxis

Hershko AY, Dranitzki Z, Ulmanski R, Levi-Schaffer F, Naparstek Y.
Clinical Immunology and Allergy Unit, Hadassah University Hospital, Jerusalem, Israel.
Scand J Clin Lab Invest. 2001; 61(6):449-52
The process underlying anaphylaxis involves an uncontrolled elevation in blood levels of mediators, including histamine. Usually, these abnormal levels are attributed to the degranulation of basophils and mast cells. Few reports have assessed the contribution of defects in histamine pharmacodynamics to allergic responses. In this report we describe a patient with recurrent anaphylaxis who was initially suspected to have enhanced histamine intolerance. We evaluated urine and blood samples collected from this patient and from control individuals using an ELISA test. Our data clearly show constitutive hyperhistaminaemia and a markedly impaired urinary histamine clearance ratio in the index patient. It is suggested that this defect facilitates anaphylaxis.

No correlation between wine intolerance and histamine content of wine

Kanny G, Gerbaux V, Olszewski A, Frémont S, Empereur F, Nabet F, Cabanis JC, Moneret-Vautrin DA.
J Allergy Clin Immunol. 2001 Feb; 107(2):375-8
BACKGROUND: Histamine is thought to be the main cause of adverse reactions to wines. OBJECTIVE: The purpose of this study was to test the hypothesis that the level of histamine in wine affects the tolerance to wine in 16 subjects with wine intolerance.
METHODS: We performed a study to examine the effects of wine histamine content in 16 adults with wine intolerance. Each subject underwent 2 double-blind provocation tests with wine: 1 with a wine poor in histamine (0.4 mg/L), and 1 with a wine rich in histamine (13.8 mg/L). Blood was collected for histamine and methylhistamine RIAs at 0, 10, 30, and 45 minutes after ingestion of the wine. Methylhistamine and methylimidazolacetic acid (gas chromatography and mass spectrometry) were measured in urine 5 hours before and 5 hours after ingestion.
RESULTS: No significant differences in the occurrence of adverse reactions were noted after ingestion of either of the wines (McNemar test). At 10 minutes, a significant increase was observed in plasma histamine with histamine-poor wine. No significant changes (Wilcoxon test) were observed in the methylhistamine and methylimidazolacetic acid levels after ingestion of either histamine-poor or histamine-rich wine.
CONCLUSION: This study demonstrates that there is no correlation between the histamine content of wine and wine intolerance. The increase of plasma histamine levels at 10 minutes with histamine-poor wine suggested the role of a histamine-releasing substance. The role of acetaldehyde is discussed.

Following the trace of elusive amines

Richard T. Premont, Raul R. Gainetdinov, and Marc G. Caron
PNAS, August 14, 2001, vol. 98, no. 17, 9474–9475

Adverse reactions to foods

Ring J, Brockow K, Behrendt H.
J Chromatogr B Biomed Sci Appl. 2001 May 25; 756(1-2):3-10
Allergic reactions to foods represent a prominent, actual and increasing problem in clinical medicine. Symptoms of food allergy comprise skin reactions (urticaria, angioedema, eczema) respiratory (bronchoconstriction, rhinitis), gastrointestinal (cramping, diarrhea) and cardiovascular symptoms with the maximal manifestation of anaphylactic shock. They can be elicited by minute amounts of allergens. The diagnosis of food allergy is done by history, skin test, in vitro allergy diagnosis and--if necessary--oral provocation tests, if possible placebo-controlled. Avoidance of respective allergens for the allergic patient, however, is often complicated or impossible due to deficits in declaration regulations in many countries. Increasing numbers of cases including fatalities, due to inadvertent intake of food allergens are reported. It is therefore necessary to improve declaration laws and develop methods for allergen detection in foods. Allergens can be detected by serological methods (enzyme immunoassays, in vitro basophil histamine release or in vivo skin test procedures in sensitized individuals). The problem of diagnosis of food allergy is further complicated by cross-reactivity between allergens in foods and aeroallergens (pollen, animal epithelia, latex etc.). Elicitors of pseudo-allergic reactions with similar clinical symptomatology comprise low-molecular-mass chemicals (preservatives, colorings, flavor substances etc.). For some of them (e.g. sulfites) detection

assays are available. In some patients classic allergic contact eczema can be elicited systemically after oral intake of low-molecular-mass contact allergens such as nickel sulfate or flavorings such as vanillin in foods. The role of xenobiotic components in foods (e.g. pesticides) is not known at the moment. In order to improve the situation of the food allergic patient, research programs to elucidate the pathophysiology and improve allergen detection strategies have to be implemented together with reinforced declaration regulations on a quantitative basis.

[Food allergy in the chronic alcoholic and alcohol in food allergy: apropos of 38 cases] [Article in French]
Serghini-Idrissi N, Ravier I, Aucouturier H, Ait Tahar H, Sonneville A.
Allerg Immunol (Paris). 2001 Dec; 33(10):378-82
Exacerbation or appearance of hypersensitivity of food origin in chronic alcoholics appears to be linked to a basis of catabolism of histamine, a facilitation of penetration of allergens under the impetus of the mucosa-irritating power of alcohol and its potential as a histamine-liberator; it results frequently in an elevated total IgE that predisposes to conflictual sub-cutaneous mechanisms, so explaining the easy appearance or exacerbation of food allergies. We have used skin tests of the principal food allergens to evaluate the influence of alcohol in the development of allergies, by determining the allergy profile of each patient and consequently, the titres of total IgE. Our results show the potentiating role in the physiopathology of allergy and food intolerance without which it helps as much by an evident inducing role in the appearance of true food allergy.

Outcome of a Histamine-restricted Diet Based on Chart Audit
Vickerstaff Joneja JM, Carmona-Silva C
Journal of Nutritional and Environmental Medicine, 2001, Vol. 11, No. 4: Pages 249-262
PURPOSE: This is a report of the outcome of dietary management (histamine restriction) of 44 subjects referred to a food allergy clinic over a 12-month period for management of 'idiopathic' urticaria, angioedema and pruritus (U/A/P), because their symptoms had resisted previous treatment and because a preliminary study had shown potential response to such a diet in comparison with placebo. Additionally, the effect of this type of dietary management was reported on numerous other symptoms.
DESIGN: Statistical evaluation of outcome based on clinical signs and symptoms.
MATERIALS AND METHODS: Because the U/A/P symptoms of the subjects evaluated in the study were characteristic of a histamine mediator response, a histamine-restricted diet was implemented for a 4-week trial. By means of chart audit, symptoms which had been rated by subjects according to severity were compared at the beginning and the end of the trial period, as was the change in intake of antihistamine medication.
RESULTS: The degree of improvement in symptoms varied, depending on the symptom reported and the gender and age of the subject. For U/A/P symptoms, 61.4% reported significant improvement, 18.2% reported 'some improvement', while 20.4% showed no improvement. Women (more prevalent) reported a greater degree of improvement than men. Of the additional symptoms, no-one reported improvement in atopic dermatitis or contact dermatitis (n = 4); 50% of subjects reported improvement in migraine headaches, while 50% reported no improvement (n = 10); 80% of subjects with gastrointestinal tract symptoms reported improvement (n = 9); 100% of subjects reporting 'panic attacks' as one of their additional problems (n = 3) reported complete remission of this symptom.
CONCLUSIONS: A randomized, double-blind controlled trial with an appropriate sample size would be required to ensure that the observed symptom relief in our subjects with recalcitrant idiopathic U/A/P is not due to bias or chance. Considering that a histamine-restricted diet has been beneficial in this uncontrolled pilot study, a time-limited trial on the diet, which poses no risk of nutritional deficiency, may be warranted for subjects exhibiting the type of resistant symptoms reported.

Benefits of a Histamine-Reducing Diet for Some Patients with Chronic Urticaria and Angioedema
WENDY King, LINDA McCargar, JANICE Joneja, SUSAN Barr
Can J Diet Pract Res. 2000; 61 (1):24-26
Urticaria and angioedema symptoms result primarily from the physiological actions of histamine. Some individuals with urticaria have a decreased ability to degrade dietary histamine before it enters the circulation. Foods high in histamine, such as fermented foods, may exacerbate urticaria and angioedema in these individuals. Certain food additives may increase endogenous release of histamine and urticaria and angioedema symptoms. The objective of this study was to evaluate the effect of a histamine-reducing diet on urticaria and angioedema symptoms, and on nutrient intake. Nineteen subjects with chronic urticaria or angioedema were randomized to a treatment group (n=9) or a control group (n=10). The treatment group followed a histamine-reducing diet, and the control group eliminated artificial sweeteners from their diets. The subjects recorded antihistamine medication intake, number of wheals, the severity of pruritus and the severity of angioedema for two weeks before starting the diet and for six weeks during the dietary intervention. Subjects completed three-day food records every two weeks. There was a marginally significant decrease in the number of

antihistamine tablets taken in the histamine-reducing diet group compared with the control group, and two of nine treatment subjects had dramatically improved symptoms. During the study there was no significant risk of nutritional deficiency for either group.

Are adverse effects of sildenafil also caused by inhibition of diamine oxidase?

Wantke F, Hemmer W, Focke M, Stackl W, Götz M, Jarisch R.

Urol Int. 2001; 67(1):59-61

BACKGROUND: Sildenafil citrate (Viagra), a drug used to treat erectile dysfunctions, causes adverse reactions such as headache, flushing or nasal congestion. Sildanefil's potency as inhibitor of diamine oxidase was investigated, as side effects may also be induced by histamine itself due to an impaired histamine metabolism.

METHODS: Placental diamine oxidase inhibition experiments were performed with consecutive dilutions of sildenafil citrate (10(-5) to 10(-9) mol/l). In 9 male volunteers in vivo diamine oxidase inhibition was investigated after taking 100 mg sildenafil (Viagra). RESULTS: Sildenafil citrate did not inhibit placental diamine oxidase either in vitro or in vivo. However, infusion of 300 mg of cimetidine inhibited diamine oxidase activity by 27 +/- 7% 15 min after infusion, demonstrating that drugs may inhibit diamine oxidase in vivo.

CONCLUSION: As side effects of sildenafil are not caused due to inhibition of diamine oxidase, sildenafil citrate seems to be harmless for patients suffering from histamine intolerance.

2000

Diet and sex-hormone binding globulin, dysmenorrhea, and premenstrual symptoms

Barnard ND, Scialli AR, Hurlock D, Bertron P.

Obstet Gynecol. 2000 Feb;95(2):245-50

OBJECTIVE: To test the hypothesis that a low-fat, vegetarian diet reduces dysmenorrhea and premenstrual symptoms by its effect on serum sex-hormone binding globulin concentration and estrogen activity.

METHODS: In a crossover design, 33 women followed a low-fat, vegetarian diet for two menstrual cycles. For two additional cycles, they followed their customary diet while taking a supplement placebo pill. Dietary intake, serum sex-hormone binding globulin concentration, body weight, pain duration and intensity, and premenstrual symptoms were assessed during each study phase.

RESULTS: Mean (+/- standard deviation [SD]) serum sex-hormone binding globulin concentration was higher during the diet phase (46.7 +/- 23.6 nmol/L) than during the supplement phase (39.3 +/- 19.8 nmol/L, P < .001). Mean (+/- SD) body weight was lower during the diet (66.1 +/- 11.3 kg) compared with the supplement phase (67.9 +/- 12.1 kg, P < .001). Mean dysmenorrhea duration fell significantly from baseline (3.9 +/- 1.7 days) to diet phase (2.7 +/- 1.9 days) compared with change from baseline to supplement phase (3.6 +/- 1.7 days, P < .01). Pain intensity fell significantly during the diet phase, compared with baseline, for the worst, second-worst, and third-worst days, and mean durations of premenstrual concentration, behavioral change, and water retention symptoms were reduced significantly, compared with the supplement phase.

CONCLUSION: A low-fat vegetarian diet was associated with increased serum sex-hormone binding globulin concentration and reductions in body weight, dysmenorrhea duration and intensity, and premenstrual symptom duration. The symptom effects might be mediated by dietary influences on estrogen activity.

Histamine plasma levels and elimination diet in chronic idiopathic urticaria

Guida B, De Martino CD, De Martino SD, Tritto G, Patella V, Trio R, D'Agostino C, Pecoraro P, D'Agostino L.

Eur J Clin Nutr. 2000 Feb; 54(2):155-8

OBJECTIVE: The aim of this study was to evaluate the effects of an oligoantigenic and histamine-free diet on patients affected with chronic idiopathic urticaria (CIU).

DESIGN: Ten patients with chronic idiopathic urticaria were prescribed an oligoantigenic and histamine-free diet for 21 days, followed by serial and controlled reintroduction of foods during a further 70 days. Modification in clinical illness as well as histamine plasma levels, post-heparin plasma diamine oxidase (DAO) and intestinal permeability were evaluated.

RESULTS: The oligoantigenic and histamine-free diet induced a significant improvement of symptoms (P<0.05). Moreover, CIU patients on free diet showed higher histamine plasma levels (P<0. 05 vs post-diet and vs controls) that fell to control levels during the oligoantigenic and histamine-free diet. Post-heparin plasma diamine oxidase values were slightly reduced and were unchanged during the diet as well as intestinal permeability, which was always normal in all patients.

CONCLUSIONS: These data suggest that histamine plays a major role in chronic idiopathic urticaria. The finding of normal intestinal permeability suggests that a morphological damage of intestinal mucosa should be excluded in these patients. However, the presence of low levels of post-heparin plasma diamine oxidase may indicate a subclinical impairment of small bowel enterocyte function that could induce a higher sensitivity to histamine-rich or histamine-producing food.

Benefits of a Histamine-Reducing Diet for Some Patients with Chronic Urticaria and Angioedema
King W, McCargar L, Joneja JM, Barr SI
Can J Diet Pract Res. 2000 Spring; 61(1):24-26

Urticaria and angioedema symptoms result primarily from the physiological actions of histamine. Some individuals with urticaria have a decreased ability to degrade dietary histamine before it enters the circulation. Foods high in histamine, such as fermented foods, may exacerbate urticaria and angioedema in these individuals. Certain food additives may increase endogenous release of histamine and urticaria and angioedema symptoms. The objective of this study was to evaluate the effect of a histamine-reducing diet on urticaria and angioedema symptoms, and on nutrient intake. Nineteen subjects with chronic urticaria or angioedema were randomized to a treatment group (n=9) or a control group (n=10). The treatment group followed a histamine-reducing diet, and the control group eliminated artificial sweeteners from their diets. The subjects recorded antihistamine medication intake, number of wheals, the severity of pruritus and the severity of angioedema for two weeks before starting the diet and for six weeks during the dietary intervention. Subjects completed three-day food records every two weeks. There was a marginally significant decrease in the number of antihistamine tablets taken in the histamine-reducing diet group compared with the control group, and two of nine treatment subjects had dramatically improved symptoms. During the study there was no significant risk of nutritional deficiency for either group.

1999

Enteral histaminosis: Clinical implications
Amon U, Bangha E, Küster T, Menne A, Vollrath IB, Gibbs BF.
Inflamm Res. 1999 Jun; 48(6):291-5

There is increasing evidence that enteral histaminosis is a major cause of food intolerance resulting from dysfunctional metabolism of endogenous histamine in certain food stuffs. However, this phenomenon has been poorly characterised and, due to the lack of epidemiological data, the existence of this condition has been underestimated, which may lead to incorrect diagnosis. This short commentary highlights a stricter regimen of diagnostic procedure in order to take into account the many causes of food intolerance. The underlying mechanisms ascribed particularly to non-immunologically food reactions require more rigorous research and further work is vital.

Biogenic amines in foods: histamine and food processing
Bodmer S, Imark C, Kneubühl M.
Inflamm Res. 1999 Jun; 48(6):296-300

Biogenic amines, e.g. histamine, occur in many different foods. At high concentrations, they are risk factors for food intoxication, whereas moderate levels may lead to food intolerance. Sensitive persons, with insufficient diamine oxidase activity, suffer from numerous undesirable reactions after intake of histamine containing foods. Besides spoiled foodstuffs, especially fermented foods tend to contain elevated levels of biogenic amines, although their concentrations vary extensively not only between different food varieties but also within the varieties themselves. High histamine content in foods and beverages result from microbial contamination. The evidence of enteral histaminosis represents a challenge for the food industry to produce foods with histamine levels as low as possible. We therefore investigated critical steps for histamine formation during food production processes, and established production methods that include low-histamine technology.

Role of food allergy and food intolerance in recurrent urticaria
Jarisch R, Beringer K, Hemmer W.
Curr Probl Dermatol. 1999; 28:64-73

Histamine content does not influence the tolerance of wine in normal subjects
Kanny G, Bauza T, Frémont S, Guillemin F, Blaise A, Daumas F, Cabanis JC, Nicolas JP, Moneret-Vautrin DA.
Allerg Immunol (Paris). 1999 Feb; 31(2):45-8

Histamine has been incriminated as having a responsibility for intolerance reaction to wines. We have made a study by double blind oral provocation test to find the effect of ingestion of a histamine-rich (22.8 mg.l-1) and a histamine free wine in eight healthy subjects. Blood samples were taken at 0, 10, 30 and 45 minutes after ingestion of the wine for measurement of plasma histamine and methylhistamine. Urines were collected 5 hours before and 5 hours after ingestion for measurement of urinary methylhistamine. No subject presented a reaction of intolerance after ingestion of wine rich or poor in histamine. No change in plasma histamine and plasma and urinary methylhistamine was seen. This study shows that the amount of histamine in wine has no clinical or biological effect in healthy subjects, and this emphasized the efficiency in man of the systems for degradation of histamine that is absorbed by the alimentary tract.

Histamine intolerance imitated a fish allergy
Thewes M, Rakoski J, Ring J.
Acta Derm Venereol. 1999 Jan; 79(1):89

Alcohol-histamine interactions
Zimatkin SM, Anichtchik OV.
Alcohol Alcohol. 1999; 34(2): 141-7
Alcohol and histamine metabolic pathways in the body have the common enzymes aldehyde dehydrogenase and aldehyde oxidase. The metabolite of ethanol, acetaldehyde, can effectively compete with the metabolites of histamine, methylimidazole acetaldehyde, and imidazole acetaldehyde. At the periphery, alcohol and acetaldehyde liberate histamine from its store in mast cells and depress histamine elimination by inhibiting diamine oxidase, resulting in elevated histamine levels in tissues. Histamine mediates alcohol-induced gastric and intestinal damage and bronchial asthma as well as flushing in Orientals. On the other hand, alcohol provokes food-induced histaminosis and histamine intolerance, which is an epidemiological problem. There are many controversial reports concerning the effect of H2 receptor antagonists on ethanol metabolism and the activity of alcohol dehydrogenase in the stomach. In addition, alcohol affects histamine levels in the brain by modulating histamine synthesis, release, and turnover. Histamine receptor antagonists can affect ethanol metabolism and change the sensitivity of animals to the hypnotic effects of alcohol. In contrast to other neurotransmitters, the involvement of the brain histamine system in the mechanisms of the central actions of alcohol and in the pathogenesis of alcoholism is poorly studied and understood.

1998

[Intolerance reaction caused by biogenic amines. A separate disease entity?][Article in German]
Bischoff SC, Manns MP.
Internist (Berl). 1998 Mar; 39(3):317-8

Beneficial effects of Helicobacter pylori eradication on migraine
Gasbarrini A, De Luca A, Fiore G, Gambrielli M, Franceschi F, Ojetti V, Torre ES, Gasbarrini G, Pola P, Giacovazzo M
Hepatogastroenterology. 1998; 45(21): 765-70
BACKGROUND/AIMS: Migraine is a commonly unilateral throbbing headache, which has been associated with disorders of the vascular tone. Helicobacter pylori, the most relevant cause of gastritis and peptic ulcer, has been recently associated with a typical functional vascular disorder such as primary Raynaud phenomenon. The aim of this study was to assess the prevalence of H. pylori for patients affected by migraine and the effects of H. pylori eradication on migraine symptoms.
METHODOLOGY: Two-hundred and twenty-five patients were consecutively enrolled between October 1996 and January 1997. H. pylori was assessed by 13C-urea breath test. Infected subjects were eradicated of the bacterium; frequency, intensity and duration of attacks of migraine were assessed during a 6 month follow-up period.
RESULTS: H. pylori was detected in 40% of the patients. Eighty-three percent of the patients who underwent therapy were eradicated. Intensity, duration and frequency of attacks of migraine were significantly reduced in all eradicated patients.
CONCLUSIONS: H. pylori is common in subjects with migraine. Bacterium eradication causes a significant decrease in attacks of migraine. The reduction of vasoactive substances produced during infection may be the pathogenetic mechanism underlying the phenomen

Human histamine N-methyltransferase pharmacogenetics: common genetic polymorphisms that alter activity
Preuss CV, Wood TC, Szumlanski CL, Raftogianis RB, Otterness DM, Girard B, Scott MC, Weinshilboum RM
Mol Pharmacol. 1998, 53(4): 708-17
Histamine N-methyltransferase (HNMT) catalyzes a major pathway in histamine metabolism. Levels of HNMT activity in humans are regulated by inheritance. We set out to study the molecular basis for this genetic regulation. Northern blot analysis showed that HNMT is highly expressed in the kidney, so we determined levels of enzyme activity and thermal stability in 127 human renal biopsy samples. DNA was isolated from 12 kidney samples with widely different HNMT phenotypes, and exons of the HNMT gene were amplified with the polymerase chain reaction. In these 12 samples, we observed a C314T transition that resulted in a Thr105Ile change in encoded amino acid, as well as an A939G transition within the 3'-untranslated region. All remaining renal biopsy samples then were genotyped for these two variant sequences. Frequencies of the alleles encoding Thr105 and Ile105 in the 114 samples studied were 0.90 and 0.10, respectively, whereas frequencies for the nucleotide A939 and G alleles

were 0.79 and 0.21, respectively. Kidney samples with the allele encoding Ile105 had significantly lower levels of HNMT activity and thermal stability than did those with the allele that encoded Thr105. These observations were confirmed by transient expression in COS-1 cells of constructs that contained all four alleles for these two polymorphisms. COS-1 cells transfected with the Ile105 allele had significantly lower HNMT activity and immunoreactive HNMT protein than did those transfected with the Thr105 allele. These observations will make it possible to test the hypothesis that genetic polymorphisms for HNMT may play a role in the pathophysiology of human disease.

Daily variations of serum diamine oxidase and the influence of H1 and H2 blockers: a critical approach to routine diamine oxidase assessment
Wantke F, Proud D, Siekierski E, Kagey-Sobotka A.
Inflamm Res. 1998 Oct; 47(10):396-400
OBJECTIVE AND DESIGN: Histamine in food has been shown to induce intolerance reactions mimicking food allergy. These reactions seem to be due to impaired histamine metabolism caused by reduced diamine oxidase activity. To validate routine serum diamine oxidase assessment, daily variations of diamine oxidase were evaluated.
METHODS: Blood was drawn from each of 20 healthy volunteers (10 female, 10 male; mean age 32.5 years) every 2 h from 9 a.m. to 5 p.m., and diamine oxidase activity was measured using the C14 putrescine method. To assess possible influences of H1 and H2 blockers on diamine oxidase activity, diphenhydramine, ketotifen, cimetidine, and ranitidine were incubated at pharmacologic concentrations with human placental diamine oxidase (identical to neutrophilic and eosinophilic diamine oxidase). Inhibition of diamine oxidase activity was calculated as the percentage of inhibition versus control. In addition, the known diamine oxidase inhibitors, dihydralazine and aminoguanidine, were used as positive controls.
RESULTS: Serum diamine oxidase levels showed no significant daily variations (0.041 +/- 0.025; 0.037 +/- 0.022; 0.041 +/- 0.023; 0.040 +/- 0.023; 0.038 +/- 0.025 nKat/l) and no significant sex differences (female 0.040 +/- 0.028 nKat/l versus male 0.039 +/- 0.019 nKat/l). Antihistamines had no influence on diamine oxidase activity except for cimetidine, which caused 25% inhibition at the highest dose tested (p < 0.0002) (positive control: aminoguanidine 85% inhibition (p< 0.0001), dihydralazine 68% inhibition (p<0.0001)) and diphenhydramine, which caused 19% increase (p<0.0001)of enzyme activity.
CONCLUSION: Serum diamine oxidase levels do not show daily variations allowing assessment anytime during office hours. However, diagnostic interpretation of serum diamine oxidase levels may be difficult.

1997

Histamine containing food: establishment of a German Food Intolerance Databank (NFID)
Diel E, Bayas N, Stibbe A, Müller S, Bott A, Schrimpf D, Diel F.
Inflamm Res. 1997 Mar; 46 Suppl 1:S87-8

1996

Biogene Amine in der Ernährung
Beutling D.M.
Springer Berlin, 1996, 265 pages, ISBN: 978-3-540-60398-6

Study to investigate the difference in reaction to intracutaneously and orally administered histamine between suspected histamine-intolerant patients and healthy volunteers
[Onderzoek naar de effecten van histamine op gezonde vrijwilligers en histamine-intolerante patienten]
Broeder E den, Kortboyer JM, Koers WJ, Bruijnzeel-Koomen CAFM, Haan-Brand A de, Wolthers BG, Breukelman H, Meulenbelt J
RIVM Rapport 348801008, 98 p, in English
A study, designed as a double-blind placebo controlled comparative study, has been performed in order to investigate the difference in reaction to intracutaneously and orally administered histamine between patients and healthy volunteers based on the assumption that histamine-intolerant patients have a relative shortage of the enzyme diamine-oxidase (DAO). Several parameters were determined in patients and compared to those in healthy volunteers. No statistical significant differences were found between patients and healthy volunteers after intracutaneous and oral administration of histamine. It can, therefore, be concluded that neither intracutaneous nor oral administration of histamine can as yet be used as a valid test to diagnose histamine-intolerance

[Pseudo-allergies are due to histamine intolerance][Article in German]
Götz M.
Wien Med Wochenschr. 1996; 146(15):426-30

Numerous undesirable reactions to alcoholic beverages, foods, drugs and other substances are characterized by allergy-like signs and symptoms and yet show unambiguously negative allergy test results. Such persons should be assessed for evidence of histamine intolerance caused by histamine overload and/or diamine oxidase deficiency. Diamine oxidase is the main histamine degrading enzyme with a predominantly gut activity. This would explain why nutritional allergies are often primarily suspected. The clinical evidence for histamine intolerance is based on chronic headache, diarrhoea, vomiting, flush, urticaria, asthma-like symptoms, rhinitis and others. Histamine restricted food, supported if necessary by H1 antihistamine blockade are simple but highly efficacious measures as shown by us in large patient groups. Intolerance to red wine probably is the most outstanding clinical characteristic and a directed question must be included into any allergy history in order to avoid missing a very major diagnostic spectrum with good therapeutic maneuverability.

Assessment of food chemical intolerance in adult asthmatic subjects

Hodge L, Yan KY, Loblay RL.
Thorax. 1996 Aug; 51(8):805-9
BACKGROUND: Identification of food chemical intolerance in asthmatic subjects can be reliably assessed by changes in the forced expiratory volume in one second FEV1) in response to double blind, placebo controlled challenges on a strict elimination diet. However, this method is cumbersome and time consuming. A study was undertaken to determine whether changes in bronchial responsiveness to histamine following food chemical challenge without an elimination diet might be a faster, more convenient method.
METHODS: Eleven adult asthmatic subjects were challenged twice with metabisulphite, aspirin, monosodium glutamate, artificial food colours, sodium nitrite/ nitrate, 0.5% citric acid solution (placebo), and sucrose (placebo) on separate days. During the first set of challenges subjects consumed a normal diet. Bronchial responsiveness to histamine was assessed 90 minutes after each challenge. A greater than twofold increase in bronchial responsiveness was considered positive. For one month prior to and during the second set of challenges subjects followed a strict elimination diet and FEV1 was monitored during and for two hours after each challenge. A fall in FEV1 of 20% or more was considered positive.
RESULTS: Of the 77 food chemical challenges performed on an unmodified diet, 20 were positive (six placebo responses). In two subjects it was not possible to perform a histamine test after one of the chemical challenges because of poor spirometric function. Of the 77 food chemical challenges performed on an elimination diet, 11 were positive (no placebo responses). Excluding the two challenges in which there were no corresponding histamine tests, only on two occasions did the positive responses in both methods coincide, giving the unmodified diet method a sensitivity of 22%.
CONCLUSIONS: Strict dietary elimination and measurement of FEV1 after double blind food chemical challenge remains the most reliable method for the detection of food chemical intolerance in asthmatic subjects.

[Specific immunotherapy in allergies--evaluation of current status][Article in German]

Jarisch R, Hemmer W.
Wien Med Wochenschr. 1996; 146(15):422-5
Specific immunotherapy is the treatment of choice in the therapy of inhalant allergies. Application route and dose regimen, selection and quality of allergens, as well as the individual patient represent different variables of immunotherapy to be considered. Premedication by oral antihistamines is mandatory for the reduction of side effects. Histamine-intolerance represents a contraindication for immunotherapy. Specific immunotherapy is highly efficacious leading to a 50-100% reduction of symptoms in nearly 90% of patients.

Wine and headache

Jarisch R, Wantke F.
Int Arch Allergy Immunol. 1996 May; 110(1):7-12
Headache can be induced by histamine in wine in patients suffering from histamine intolerance, a disease characterized by impaired histamine degradation based on reduced diamine oxidase activity or a lack of the enzyme. Diamine oxidase is localized in the jejunal mucosa and is the most important enzyme metabolizing histamine. It is competitively inhibited by alcohol and numerous drugs. In preliminary investigations, assessment of diamine oxidase levels gave decreased activity (0.03 nKat/l) in patients with histamine intolerance compared to healthy controls (0.07 nKat/l). In pregnancy, diamine oxidase levels are known to be about 500-fold elevated, giving mean levels of 25.0 nKat/l. Other biogenic amines such as phenylethylamine or serotonin may be causative for wine/food-induced headache. In experimental models, headache has been induced by histamine infusion as well as red wine provocation. Histamine-induced headache is a vascular headache likely to be caused by nitric oxide which probably represents a key molecule in vascular headaches. A histamine-free diet is the treatment of choice for patients with histamine intolerance and chronic headache. To start treatment, an antihistamine (H1 blocker) for 14 days as well as a histamine-free diet for at least 4 weeks are recommended. Clinical improvement to the diet as well as in vitro tests for plasma histamine and

diamine oxidase in the serum as well as vitamin B6 levels have to confirm the diagnosis. As supportive treatment, a vitamin B6 (pyridoxal phosphate) substitution appears useful in histamine-intolerant patients as pyridoxal phosphate seems to be crucial for diamine oxidase activity. Histamine intolerance, based on reduced diamine oxidase activity or a lack in the enzyme is causative for wine/food-induced chronic headache. According to the localization of diamine oxidase in the jejunal mucosa, histamine intolerance is primarily a disease of intestinal origin. A histamine-free diet is the treatment of choice in histamine-intolerant patients suffering from chronic headache. In addition, it is also important to avoid diamine-oxidase-blocking drugs and alcohol which act as inhibitors of diamine oxidase. As avoidance of histamine-rich food is simple, inexpensive and harmless treatment, histamine-containing food such as cheese and alcoholic beverages should be labeled.

Ultrastructural changes in the duodenal mucosa induced by ingested histamine in patients with chronic urticaria

Kanny G, Grignon G, Dauca M, Guedenet JC, Moneret-Vautrin DA.

Allergy. 1996 Dec; 51(12):935-9

Histamine in food may be responsible for some cases of food intolerance. We previously demonstrated disturbances in the metabolism of ingested histamine in patients with chronic urticaria (CU) and proposed that this could be related to increased intestinal permeability to histamine. The present study was undertaken to look for ultrastructural changes in the intestinal tract that might explain this abnormality. We examined duodenal biopsies from seven patients with CU before and after intraduodenal administration of histamine (120 mg). Five subjects had clinical symptoms (diarrhea, urticaria, headache, accelerated heart rate, and drop in blood pressure) within 1 h of duodenal histamine challenge (DHC). Ultrastructural changes, including edema of the interstitial tissue, enlargement of the basal intercellular spaces, slight congestion of the endothelial cells, and pericapillary edema, were observed in six subjects 45 min after DHC. In all the biopsies, the epithelium was normal, and the tight junctions were not modified by DHC. This morphologic study demonstrates that histamine can induce edema in the basal intercellular spaces of the duodenal mucosa and in the submucosa without evident change in the integrity of intercellular junctions. The most plausible route for histamine to have taken would appear to be an intracellular one.

[Pseudoallergic reactions. Intolerance to natural and synthetic food constituents masquerading as food allergy][Article in Polish]

Kurek M.

Pediatr Pol. 1996 Sep;71(9):743-52

Adverse hypersensitivity reactions to natural foods and certain drugs and food additives are mediated by immunological (allergy) or non-immunological mechanisms. Some clinical and physiological similarities have been noted between these allergic and non-allergic reactions. This observation has led to the concept of "pseudoallergic reactions-PAR". PAR can be triggered in various ways such as: interactions with the central or peripherical nervous system, non-specific release of mediators, enzyme inhibition due to hereditary or pharmacologically induced enzyme deficiencies and pharmacological properties of some natural food constituents such as biogenic amines. The prevalence of adverse reactions to food additives has been calculated to be about 0.1%. PAR to food additives occurs frequently in patients suffering from urticaria, asthma and may be accompanied by history of aspirin or NSAI pseudoallergic reactions. The same additives (azo dyes, sulphites, benzoates) are used in various drug formulations and may be responsible for eliciting PAR. In Poland, labelling of food additives, following the "E number system", has been mandatory since 1993. Unfortunately, this satisfactory trend has not yet been applied to drug additives. The diagnosis of PAR to food additives is based on the anamnesis with analysis of the patient's drug and dietary intake. Skin tests and "in vitro" tests are only sporadically informative. In each individual patient, a specific challenge with additives is desirable. Food additives may be tested according to the schedule based on DBPCFC principle. Individually performed exclusion regimes are the principal methods of prevention.

[Diet and migraine]. [Article in Spanish]

Leira R, Rodríguez R

Rev Neurol. 1996; 24(129): 534-8

Some foods in our diet can spark off migraine attacks in susceptible individuals. Some foods can bring an attack on through an allergic reaction. A certain number such as citrus fruits, tea, coffee, pork, chocolate, milk, nuts, vegetables and cola drinks have been cited as possible allergens associated with migraine. This mechanism has however been criticized: an improvement in symptoms by eliminating some food(s) from our diet does not necessarily mean an immunologically based allergic reaction. The high IgE incidence rate is not greater in such patients than in the population at large. Other allergic reactions unrelated to diet may also be associated with migraine attacks. On the other hand substances in food may be the cause of modifications in vascular tone and bring migraine on in those so prone. Among such substances are tyramine, phenylalanine, phenolic flavonoids, alcohol, food additives (sodium nitrate, monosodium glutamate, aspartame) and caffeine. Another recognized trigger for migraine is hypoglycemia. Such foods as chocolate, cheese, citrus fruits, bananas, nuts, 'cured' meats, dairy products, cereals, beans, hot dogs, pizza, food additives (sodium nitrate, monosodium glutamate in Chinese restaurant food, aspartame as a sweetener), coffee, tea, cola drinks, alcoholic drinks such as red wine, beer or whisky distilled in copper stills, all may bring on a migraine attack. For every patient we have to assess which foodstuffs are involved in the attack (not necessarily produced by consuming the product concerned) in order to try to avoid their consumptions as a means of prophylaxis for migraine.

Outdoor pollution and headache

Nattero G, Enrico A.
Headache. 1996 Apr;36(4):243-5
The aim of this study was to clarify a possible relationship between pollution and worsening of headache in the industrial city of Turin. From October 1992 to June 1993, we examined a group of 32 patients suffering from various headache types. During these months, they kept a daily record of their headaches and associated disturbances. Changes in pain frequency and severity were recorded every hour of the day and compared hour to hour with the various degrees of pollution recorded in the main streets by a monitoring station. The influence of meteorological parameters was also taken into consideration. During winter, carbon monoxide and nitrogen dioxide showed a simultaneous hyperconcentration on the same days and the same hours. Increased incidence of headache attacks and increase in severity corresponded to the same hours, days, and months. The findings were statistically significant (P = 0.008, Student's t-test). An isolated increase in nitrogen dioxide only (without an increase in carbon monoxide which was only recorded once) induced headache a couple of hours after the peak concentration was reached. Among the meteorological factors, only the highest values in wind velocity were shown to exert a significant influence on worsening headache frequency and severity.

Histamine in wine. Bronchoconstriction after a double-blind placebo-controlled red wine provocation test

Wantke F, Hemmer W, Haglmüller T, Götz M, Jarisch R.
Int Arch Allergy Immunol. 1996 Aug; 110(4):397-400
A 38-year-old woman with a history of seasonal rhinoconjunctivitis reported repeated attacks of wheezing after drinking various alcoholic beverages. Two consecutive histamine provocations using two identical samples of red wine containing 200 micrograms histamine/l and 3,700 micrograms/l, respectively, were performed in a double-blind placebo-controlled fashion to assess a possible histamine-induced bronchoconstriction. Lung function, plasma histamine, skin temperature, pulse rate and symptoms were assessed. In 3 male controls, four consecutive wine tests were performed in a randomised double-blind placebo-controlled fashion. Drinking wine with 3,700 micrograms histamine/l caused coughing and wheezing with a decrease in lung function. Plasma histamine showed an increase at 10 and 20 min and decreased at 30 min both after histamine-rich as well as histamine-poor wine, reaching the peak increase after histamine-rich wine. Controls did not react and plasma histamine levels did not increase. Bronchoconstriction after wine or food rich in histamine seems to be caused by diminished histamine degradation on the basis of reduced activity of diamine oxidase. Histamine in wine may induce bronchoconstriction in patients suffering from histamine intolerance.

1995

The role of additives in chronic pseudo-allergic dermatopathies from food intolerance

Antico A, Di Berardino L.
Allerg Immunol (Paris). 1995 May; 27(5):157-60
In the vast area of qualitative pathologies caused by foods, real IgE-mediated allergic reactions are rather rare. More commonly observed and apparently on a constant rise in Western countries are reactions from food intolerance, especially in relationship with the massive exposure to additives used in industrial food products. This study involved a population of 582 adult patients with chronic pseudo-allergic dermatopathies. The link between symptoms and intolerance to food additives has been proved on the basis of the efficacy of a strict diet that eliminates certain foods and the positivity of the provocation test in double-blind trial controlled with a placebo in 165 patients (about 28% of the cases). These results lead us to conclude that additives are a frequent cause of chronic pseudo-allergic dermatopathies in adult patients and, in general, a problem of primary importance in the allergology practice.

Menstrual pain in Danish women correlated with low n-3 polyunsaturated fatty acid intake

Deutch B.
Eur J Clin Nutr. 1995 Jul;49(7):508-16
OBJECTIVES: The hypothesis tested was that menstrual discomfort, e.g. dysmenorrhoea, known to be prostaglandin-mediated, can be influenced by the dietary ratio of n-3 and n-6 polyunsaturated fatty acids. The prostaglandins derived from marine n-3 fatty acids are normally less aggressive and therefore expected to be associated with milder symptoms.

DESIGN: The question was surveyed in an epidemiological study based upon self-administered questionnaires concerning menstrual history, present symptoms, general health, socioeconomic factors, and general dietary habits. Two (prospective) 4-day dietary records were used to estimate average daily nutrient intake.

SUBJECTS: The subjects were recruited by advertising (about 220 volunteered); 181 healthy Danish women were selected, aged 20-45 years; they were not pregnant and did not use oral contraceptives.

RESULTS: No correlations were found between socioeconomic or anthropometric data and menstrual problems. On the contrary certain dietary habits, e.g. low intake of animal and fish products, and intakes of specific nutrients, were correlated with menstrual pain. The average dietary n-3/n-6 ratio of women with menstrual pain was 0.24. It was significantly higher among those with low intake of B12 coincident with low intake of n-3 (0.42, $P < 0.001$) (chi-square), with low n-3 intake coincident with low n-3/n-6 ratio (0.42, $P < 0.005$), and finally with low intake of B12 coincident with low n-3/n-6 ratio (0.47, $P < 0.001$).

CONCLUSION: The results were highly significant and mutually consistent and supported the hypothesis that a higher intake of marine n-3 fatty acids correlates with milder menstrual symptoms.

Food intolerance and allergy
Pace V.
Panminerva Med. 1995 Jun; 37(2):84-91

Various food products can trigger disagreeable symptoms in certain people which are generally described as food intolerances. Given the complexity of the subject and the fact that a great deal remains to be learned about the mechanisms esponsible for these reactions, the paper attempts to clarify the whole question. Food intolerances have been classified in various ways by different authors. The present paper considers only the three major groups: those due to enzyme deficiencies, those due to an allergic mechanism and those caused by histamine-release or histamine-releasing food products.

1994

Food allergy and food intolerance--what is the difference?
Bindslev-Jensen C, Skov PS, Madsen F, Poulsen LK.
Ann Allergy. 1994 Apr; 72(4):317-20

The literature is contradictory concerning the use (and misuse) of the terms "food allergy" and "food intolerance." When using double-blind, placebo-controlled food challenge as the gold standard, the clinical picture characterizing both diseases is identical, ie, concomitant signs and symptoms from the skin, gastrointestinal-tract and respiratory system (classical allergic signs and symptoms). A distinction between food allergy and food intolerance thus depends on whether the involvement of the immune system can be verified. The basic problem with diagnostic tests such as skin prick test (SPT), measurement of specific IgE (RAST) or histamine release from basophils (HR) is that in contrast to inhalant allergens, no standardized extracts are commercially available. It is therefore often not possible to discriminate between the ability of a test per se in the diagnosis of food allergy and differences in allergen extract quality. This is probably the reason for the great variability in diagnostic sensitivity and specificity reported in the literature. Many cases of food allergy to proteins may be therefore misdiagnosed as food intolerance due to a low sensitivity of the tests (SPT, RAST, and HR) used.

[Progress in the study of histamine liberators and their mechanisms]. [Article in Chinese]
Lin YH, Xu JH
Sheng Li Ke Xue Jin Zhan. 1994 Jan;25(1):42-7

Diamine oxidase is the amiloride-binding protein and is inhibited by amiloride analogues
Novotny WF, Chassande O, Baker M, Lazdunski M, Barbry P.
J Biol Chem. 1994 Apr 1;269(13):9921-5

Diamine oxidase (histaminase), an enzyme that oxidatively deaminates putrescine and histamine, was purified from human placenta and from pig kidney. Both NH2-terminal sequences are highly homologous to the human kidney amiloride-binding protein, previously thought to be a component of the amiloride-sensitive Na+ channel. Monoclonal antibodies raised against the pig kidney amiloride-binding protein immunoprecipitate a polypeptide with the same M(r) (105,000) as that of pig kidney diamine oxidase. That polypeptide has both diamine oxidase activity and the capacity to bind [3H]phenamil, a tritiated amiloride derivative. Cells stably transfected with human kidney amiloride-binding protein cDNA express a high diamine oxidase activity. In transfected cells as well as with the purified enzyme, this activity was inhibited by amiloride and by some of its derivatives, such as phenamil and ethylpropylamiloride. Amiloride inhibition seems to be due to drug binding at the active site of the enzyme. These data indicate that human placental diamine oxidase is identical to the human kidney amiloride-binding protein and that amiloride analogues may have wider physiological effects besides those on epithelial ion transport.

Dietary treatment of Crohn's disease
Wantke F, Götz M, Jarisch R.
Lancet. 1994 Jan 8;343(8889):113
Comment on
Treatment of active Crohn's disease by exclusion diet: East Anglian multicentre controlled trial.
[Lancet. 1993]

The red wine provocation test: intolerance to histamine as a model for food intolerance
Wantke F, Götz M, Jarisch R.
Allergy Proc. 1994 Jan-Feb; 15(1):27-32
Sneezing, flush, headache, diarrhea, skin itch, and shortness of breath are symptoms occurring in patients intolerant to wine after drinking one glass of red wine. The role of histamine in wine intolerance was evaluated by a red wine provocation test in 28 patients with a history of wine intolerance and in 10 controls with good tolerance of wine. Patients were challenged with 125 ml red wine (equivalent to 50 micrograms histamine); blood samples were drawn before and after 15 and 30 minutes. Plasma histamine was assessed by a radioimmunoassay. Lung function tests were performed before and after the wine test. Twenty-two of twenty-eight patients had symptoms showing significantly higher plasma histamine levels 30 minutes after wine challenge ($p < .01$) compared with asymptomatic controls. Basal histamine levels of patients were higher ($p < .05$) than in controls. A slight asthmatic attack as well as a 30% decrease of FEF 25 was seen in 2/22 patients. Terfenadine premedication significantly eliminated symptoms in 10/12 patients ($p < .05$) in a subsequent wine test. Histamine assessment was done in 52 wines (red, white, and champagne) and in 17 beers by radioimmunoassay. Histamine levels ranged from 3-120 micrograms/l in white wines; 15-670 micrograms/l in champagnes; 60-3800 micrograms/l in red wines; and 21-305 micrograms/l in beers. Histamine is causing wine intolerance. Patients intolerant to wine seem to have diminished histamine degradation probably based on a deficiency of diamine oxidase.

1993

[Migraine and food intolerance: a controlled study in pediatric patients][Article in Italian]
Guariso G, Bertoli S, Cernetti R, Battistella PA, Setari M, Zacchello F.
Pediatr Med Chir. 1993 Jan-Feb; 15(1):57-61
The possible correlation between migraine and food intolerance has been found to be of great interest in the recent literature. We have studied 43 patients aged from 7 to 18 years suffering from migraine without aura according to the classification of International Headache Society (IHS): they had at least 2 attacks monthly and they were pharmacological free of any prophylactic treatment for the latest three months. Each patient was given an allergologic anamnesis. Half of them (group A) were first in oligoantigenic regimen (including 8 simple foods) for 4 weeks. Afterward each patient has been challenged weekly in an open trial, introducing in the diet the different foods and additives previously eliminated; then they have been controlled in a simple double blind study. We have taken skin tests (PRICK method) for the most important allergens (foods and main inhalants), plasma levels of total and specific IgE (PRIST and RAST method), and moreover we have taken histamine plasma levels at the beginning and at the end of the oligoantigenic diet, and during challenge test, only in case of headache attacks. The second half of the patients (group B) were not following any diet nor a pharmacological prophylaxis, but they have been followed up with a clinical diary. Among the patients on oligoantigenic diet 12 only concluded the trial: 6/12 presented a completed remission of headache, 5/12 had a significant improvement of the migrainous pattern, 1/12 patients did not get any improvement after the dietetic treatment. The food recognized responsible of the attacks were: cacao, banana, egg, hazelnuts. (ABSTRACT TRUNCATED AT 250 WORDS)

Diet and migraine
Jarman J
Biogenic Amines. 1993 ; 9(5/6): 441-442

Histamine-free diet: treatment of choice for histamine-induced food intolerance and supporting treatment for chronic headaches
Wantke F, Götz M, Jarisch R.
Clin Exp Allergy. 1993 Dec; 23(12):982-5
Comment in: Clin Exp Allergy. 1993 Dec;23(12):971-2.
Histamine-induced food intolerance is not IgE-mediated. Skin-prick testing and specific IgE to food allergens are typically negative. Food rich in histamine or red wine may cause allergy-like symptoms such as sneezing, flush, skin itching, diarrhoea and even shortness of breath. The suspected reason is a diminished histamine degradation based on a deficiency of diamine oxidase. As diamine oxidase cannot be supplemented, a histamine-free diet was implemented to reduce histamine intake. Forty-five patients with a history of suffering from intolerance to food or wine (n = 17) and chronic headache (n = 28) were put on the diet over months to years. Fish, cheese, hard cured sausages,

pickled cabbage and alcoholic beverages had to be avoided. Complaint intensity and drug-use per week prior to and 4 weeks after a histamine-free diet were compared. After 4 weeks on the diet 33/45 patients improved considerably (P < 0.01), eight of them had total remission. In 12/45 patients, however, no changes in symptoms were observed. Symptoms of food or wine intolerance significantly decreased (P < 0.02; treatment of choice), headaches decreased in frequency (P < 0.001), duration and intensity. After eating histamine-rich food symptoms were reproducible and could be eliminated by anti-histamines in most patients. These data indicate the role of histamine in food and wine intolerance and that histamine-rich food causes a worsening of symptoms in patients suffering from chronic headaches. Results obtained support the hypothesis of a deficiency of diamine oxidase in patients with intolerance to food or wine.

[The histamine-free diet][Article in German]
Wantke F, Götz M, Jarisch R.
Hautarzt. 1993 Aug; 44(8):512-6
Food intolerance is not IgE-mediated but caused by histamine. A diminished histamine degradation based on a deficiency of diaminoxidase is suspected to be the reason. The therapeutic efficacy of a histamine-free diet was evaluated in 100 patients with food intolerance and allergic diseases, who were required to avoid fish, cheese, hardcured sausage, pickled cabbage, wine and beer for 4 weeks. Considerable improvement was observed in 57 patients, 15 of whom had total remission. The most striking treatment results were obtained in food or wine intolerance (80% P < 0.05; treatment of choice), bronchial asthma (80%), headache (64%) and urticaria (58%). After ingestion of food rich in histamine clearcut recurrence of atopic eczema was seen in 50% of the patients affected. Histamine plays a major part in food and wine intolerance. Histamine in food causes worsening of symptoms in atopics and patients suffering from headache. The results obtained indicate a deficiency of diaminoxidase in patients with intolerance to food or wine. Histamine levels in alcoholic beverages should be displayed on the labels.

1992

Chocolate is a migraine-provoking agent
Gibb CM, Davies PT, Glover V, Steiner TJ, Clifford Rose F, Sandler M
Cephalalgia. 1991; 11(2): 93-5
Patients with migraine who believed that chocolate could provoke their attacks were challenged with either chocolate or a closely matching placebo. In a double-blind parallel group study, chocolate ingestion was followed by a typical migraine episode in 5 out of 12 patients, while none of the 8 patients challenged with placebo had an attack (p = 0.051). The median time to the onset of the attack was 22 h. This brief study provides some objective evidence that chocolate is able to provoke a migraine attack in certain patients who believe themselves sensitive to it.

Effect of diet treatment on enuresis in children with migraine or hyperkinetic behavior
Egger J, Carter CH, Soothill JF, Wilson J.
Clin Pediatr (Phila). 1992 May; 31(5):302-7
Twenty-one children with migraine and/or hyperkinetic behavior disorder which was successfully treated with an oligoantigenic (few-foods) diet also suffered from nocturnal and/or diurnal enuresis. On diet, the enuresis stopped in 12 of these children and improved in an additional four. Identification of provoking foods was by sequential reintroduction of the foods that were avoided on the oligoantigenic diet. In eight of the 12 children who recovered on the oligoantigenic diet and in the four who improved, reintroduction of one or more foods provoked a reproducible relapse of the enuresis. Nine children were subjected to a placebo-controlled, double-blind reintroduction of provoking foods. Six children relapsed during testing with incriminated foods; none reacted to placebo. Enuresis in food-induced migraine and/or behavior disorder seems to respond, in some patients, to avoidance of provoking foods.

Histamine N-methyl transferase: inhibition by drugs
Pacifici GM, Donatelli P, Giuliani L.
Br J Clin Pharmacol. 1992 Oct;34(4):322-7
1. Histamine N-methyl transferase activity was measured in samples of human liver, brain, kidney, lung and intestinal mucosa. The mean (+/- s.d.) rate (nmol min-1 mg-1 protein) of histamine N-methylation was 1.78 +/- 0.59 (liver, n = 60), 1.15 +/- 0.38 (renal cortex, n = 8), 0.79 +/- 0.14 (renal medulla, n = 8), 0.35 +/- 0.08 (lung, n = 20), 0.47 +/- 0.18 (human intestine, n = 30) and 0.29 +/- 0.14 (brain, n = 13).
2. Inhibition of histamine N-methyl transferase by 15 drugs was investigated in human liver. The IC50 for the various drugs ranged over three orders of magnitude; chloroquine was the most potent inhibitor.
3. The average IC50 values for chloroquine were 12.6, 22.0, 19.0, 21.6 microM in liver, renal cortex, brain and colon, respectively. These values are lower than the Michaelis-Menten constant for

histamine N-methyltransferase in liver (43.8 microM) and kidney (45.5 microM). Chloroquine carried a mixed non-competitive inhibition of hepatic histamine N-methyl transferase. Some side-effects of chloroquine may be explained by inhibition of histamine N-methyl transferase.

1991

The importance of endogenous histamine relative to dietary histamine in the aetiology of scombrotoxicosis
Ijomah P, Clifford MN, Walker R, Wright J, Hardy R, Murray CK
Food Addit Contam. 1991 Jul-Aug;8(4):531-42
Deliberately spoiled mackerel samples and mackerel samples implicated in outbreaks of scombrotoxicosis were, under medical supervision, tested blind on normal, healthy volunteers of both sexes. These experiments identified batches of fish which could induce nausea/vomiting and/or diarrhoea when 50 g samples were consumed. It was also established that the fillets in a batch were neither of equal potency nor homogeneous with respect to histamine content. Strong evidence was obtained that dietary histamine is not a major determinant of scombrotoxicosis since potency was not positively correlated with the dose, and volunteers appeared to fall into susceptible and non-susceptible subgroups. However, there is no reason to suspect allergy as being solely responsible for these differences in sensitivity. It is also possible to discount body weight as a factor. While the data suggest that females may be more susceptible than males, this effect cannot be confirmed at the present time. Studies with susceptible volunteers predosed with either placebo or H1 antagonist (chlorpheniramine 4 mg) demonstrated convincingly that the antihistamine can abolish vomiting and diarrhoea associated with the ingestion of 50 g of scombrotoxic fish. It is therefore postulated that endogenous histamine released by mast cell degranulation has a significant role in the aetiology of scombrotoxicosis, whereas the role of dietary histamine is minor. The nature and origin of the agent responsible for mast cell degranulation is being investigated.

Evidence that histamine is the causative toxin of scombroid-fish poisoning
Morrow JD, Margolies GR, Rowland J, Roberts LJ
N Engl J Med. 1991 Mar 14; 324(11):716-20
BACKGROUND:
The highest morbidity worldwide from fish poisoning results from the ingestion of spoiled scombroid fish, such as tuna and mackerel, and its cause is not clear. Histamine could be responsible, because spoiled scombroid fish contain large quantities of histamine. Whether histamine is the causative toxin, however, has remained in question. To address this issue, we investigated whether histamine homeostasis is altered in poisoned people.
METHODS:
The urinary excretion of histamine and its metabolite, N-methylhistamine, was measured in three persons who had scombroid-fish poisoning (scombrotoxism) after the ingestion of marlin. We measured 9 alpha, 11 beta-dihydroxy-15-oxo-2,3,18,19-tetranorprost-5-ene-1,20-dioic acid (PGD-M), the principal metabolite of prostaglandin D2, a mast-cell secretory product, to assess whether mast cells had been activated to release histamine.
RESULTS:
The fish contained high levels of histamine (842 to 2503 mumol per 100 g of tissue). Symptoms of scombrotoxism--flushing and headache--began 10 to 30 minutes after the ingestion of fish. In urine samples collected one to four hours after fish ingestion, the levels of histamine and N-methylhistamine were 9 to 20 times and 15 to 20 times the normal mean, respectively. During the subsequent 24 hours, the levels fell to 4 to 15 times and 4 to 11 times the normal values. Levels of both were normal 14 days later. PGD-M excretion was not increased at any time. Two persons treated with diphenhydramine had prompt amelioration of symptoms.
CONCLUSIONS:
Scombroid-fish poisoning is associated with urinary excretion of histamine in quantities far exceeding those required to produce toxicity. The histamine is most likely derived from the spoiled fish. These results identify histamine as the toxin responsible for scombroid-fish poisoning.

1990

[Food allergies and pseudo-allergies--mechanism, clinical aspects and diagnosis] [Article in German]
Gailhofer G, Soyer HP, Ludvan M.
Wien Med Wochenschr. 1990 May 15; 140(9):227-32
Allergic and pseudoallergic reactions caused by foods respectively food-additives present cutaneous (urticaria, erythrodermia), gastrointestinal (nausea, vomiting, diarrhoea) and respiratory symptoms (allergic bronchial asthma). The anaphylactic shock is the most severe manifestation. Exact diagnosis is based on anamnesis, skin-tests, laboratory investigations, dietetic test procedures and oral provocation. In allergic and pseudoallergic reactions the adequate therapy is the avoidance of the causative agent (diet).

Diamine oxidase activities in the large bowel mucosa of ulcerative colitis patients

Mennigen R, Kusche J, Streffer C, Krakamp B.

Agents Actions. 1990 Apr;30(1-2):264-6

The term colitis suggests mucosal inflammation as the key event. However, it may be that the disease starts with mucosal hyperproliferation, and inflammation of the impaired mucosa is a succeeding event. Therefore we studied the activity of the intestinal diamine oxidase (DAO) in ulcerative colitis (UC). This enzyme was shown to have a mucosal antiproliferative function. Biopsy specimens of 30 patients having a normal rectosigmoidal mucosa showed a DAO activity of 22.8 nmol/min g. In 12 UC patients the DAO activity was 2.7 nmol/min g (p = 0.01). In 3 patients where UC was in remission the DAO activity was 103, 107 and 208 nmol/min g, indicating an antiproliferative rebound effect. Together with the strongly reduced monoamine oxidase (MAO) activity, the decrease in DAO activity indicates that the large bowel in UC is unable to produce a proliferation terminating substance (probably gamma-aminobutyrate) derived from polyamine metabolism by oxidative deamination (DAO) or by the interconversion pathway (MAO).

Intestinal diamine oxidases and enteral-induced histaminosis: studies on three prognostic variables in an epidemiological model

Sattler J, Lorenz W

J Neural Transm Suppl, 1990; 32: 291–314

The danger of luminal histamine administered orally or formed in the intestinal fluid by bacteria has long been neglected. However, the demonstration of blocking intestinal diamine oxidase (DAO) by a variety of common drugs has revived the discussion and has created a new disease concept: enteral-induced histaminosis. In an animal model the three central prognostic variables of this disease concept (large amounts of histamine in food to make the individual ill, blocking of DAO by commonly used drugs, and the relationship between increased plasma histamine levels and disease manifestation by exogenous histamine application) were tested with randomized trials in vivo and biochemical tests in vitro using semipurified enzymes from pig and man. In the first trials authentic histamine in quantities similar to that in normal amounts of food or cheese bought from a supermarket produced life-threatening reactions if the DAO was inhibited by pretreatment with aminoguanidine. In the second series of experiments in vitro a numerous commonly used drugs was shown to inhibit both the porcine and human enzyme. Some of the inhibitors were really strong, such as dihydralazine, chloroquine, pentamidine, cycloserine, clavulanic acid, dobutamine, pancuronium and others. The type of inhibition was sometimes competitive as in the case of dihydralazine and pancuronium, sometimes non competitive (e.g. pentamidine) which may be important for long-term treatment. In the third group of experiments a relationship between the dose of i.v. injected histamine and the elevation in plasma histamine levels and clinical symptoms in pigs was demonstrated. Hence, elevated plasma histamine in pigs acts as a pathogenetic factor for the disease manifestation. It is concluded that after modelling enteral-induced histaminosis in an animal the trias of variables shown in this study should be consequently investigated in man.

Human intestinal diamine oxidase (DAO) activity in Crohn's disease: a new marker for disease assessment?

Schmidt WU, Sattler J, Hesterberg R, Röher HD, Zoedler T, Sitter H, Lorenz W.

Agents Actions. 1990 Apr;30(1-2):267-70

The key-enzyme for the metabolism of diamines in man is diamine oxidase (DAO). Its highest activities are in the intestinal mucosa, localized in the cytoplasm of the mature enterocytes of the small and large bowel. If the gut is affected by inflammation in Crohn's disease macroscopical changes are observed. This prospective study investigated if these mucosal alterations are also reflected in changes of mucosal diamine oxidase activity and/or mucosal histamine content respectively. Twenty patients (12 female, 8 male; age: means = 31, range 18-49 years) undergoing gut resection because of complications in Crohn's disease (Jan.-Dec. 1988) formed the basis of the study. Tissue samples of the resected material from areas inflamed and histologically not involved in the disease were investigated for diamine oxidase activities and histamine content. Diamine oxidase activities in the mucosa obtained from the macroscopically normal proximal (155.6; (76-393) mU/g (means, range)) and distal (132; (58.5-295) mU/g) resection margins were similar to our previous findings. In all patients, however, samples from the diseased mucosa had significantly (ca. 50%) lower diamine oxidase activities (74.5; (5-262) mU/g) compared to the healthy tissue. Similar differences were found in material obtained either from whole intestinal wall or from the mucosa. The determination of diamine oxidase activity constitutes possibly a more unambiguous and earlier parameter for assessing the extent of the inflamed area than histological disease presentations. Using biopsies the necessary extent of resection could be estimated before operation: this may influence operative strategies and help in the definition of the minimum amount of inflamed gut to be removed.

1989

Studies with volunteers on the role of histamine in suspected scombrotoxicosis
Clifford MN, Walker R, Wright J, Hardy R, Murray CK
Journal of the Science of Food and Agriculture, 1989, 47/3, 365–375
The results are reported of single-blind, medically supervised studies in volunteers of the association between the histamine content of mackerel and the incidence of scombrotoxicosis. Volunteers consumed 25 or 50 g of fresh or spoiled mackerel containing varying quantities of endogenous or added histamine. In one study the ability of HI and H2 histamine antagonists to modify symptoms was investigated. Objective parameters (pulse rate, skin temperature and peak expiratory flow rate) were recorded for 6 h, and subjective parameters (headache, flushing, oral tingling, visual disturbances, abdominal pain, nausea, palpitations, wheeziness, diarrhoea, flatulence, shivering and miscellaneous) for 24 h. No significant effects were observed, even with portions of spoiled mackerel containing 300 mg histamine, or mackerel from a batch which was reported to have been associated with an incident diagnosed as scombrotoxicosis.
It is concluded that the precise combination of circumstances required to cause a scombrotoxic event were not reproduced in these studies, but it is tentatively concluded that histamine alone is unlikely to be the causative agent.

1988

Inhibition of histamine N-methyltransferase activity in guinea-pig pulmonary alveolar macrophages by nicotine
Gairola C, Godin CS, Houdi AA, Crooks PA
J Pharm Pharmacol. 1988 Oct;40(10):724-6
Both S-(-)- and R-(+)-nicotine enantiomers are inhibitors of histamine N tau-methylation activity in guinea-pig pulmonary alveolar macrophage cultures, exhibiting IC50 values of 7 and 8 microM, respectively. S-(-)-Nicotine is not biotransformed under the conditions of the experiment, however, R-(+)-nicotine undergoes significant N-methylation to produce N-methylnicotinium ion. S-(-)-Nicotine appears to inhibit the N-methylation of its optical antipode by the alveolar nicotine N-methyltransferase. The results indicate that a contributing factor in the toxicology of cigarette smoke inhalation may be due to the inhibition of pulmonary metabolism of histamine by nicotine.

Vecuronium inhibits histamine N-methyltransferase
Futo J, Kupferberg JP, Moss J, Fahey MR, Cannon JE, Miller RD.
Anesthesiology. 1988 Jul;69(1):92-6
Although there have been clinical reports of significant hypotension and flushing associated with the use of vecuronium, it produces minimal cardiovascular effects in the vast majority of patients. In addition, there is no evidence that vecuronium stimulates the release of histamine. The authors performed in vitro kinetic studies to determine the effect of vecuronium on histamine N-methyltransferase (HNMT), the primary catabolic enzyme for histamine in humans. They also examined plasma from patients who had received vecuronium (0.1 or 0.2 mg/kg) to determine whether clinically used concentrations of the drug could inhibit HNMT. It was determined that vecuronium is a strong inhibitor of HNMT; apparent Ki = 1 microM. The inhibition is competitive with respect to methyl-donor and noncompetitive with respect to histamine. Vecuronium, in doses greater than or equal to 0.1 mg/kg, may delay the metabolism of histamine by HNMT in vitro.

Food-induced histaminosis as an epidemiological problem: plasma histamine elevation and haemodynamic alterations after oral histamine administration and blockade of diamine oxidase (DAO)
Sattler J, Häfner D, Klotter HJ, Lorenz W, Wagner PK.
Agents Actions 1988; 23(3-4): 361–5
In a randomized controlled trial, 30 pigs were orally treated with histamine (60 mg). In addition, half of the animals underwent a specific blockade of the enzyme diamine oxidase (DAO), which is the main histamine catabolising enzyme in the intestinal tract. Only these DAO-blocked animals exhibited severe clinical symptoms (e.g. hypotension, flush, vomiting) and, in parallel, showed tremendous elevations of plasma histamine levels of up to 160 ng/ml. 3 out of 15 animals in this group died within the experimental period. In contrast, the control animals neither exhibited plasma histamine levels above 5 ng/ml nor had any clinical reactions. These results contradict the current opinion that oral histamine intake in food is not clinically relevant, especially since many commonly used drugs are DAO-inhibitors and approximately 20% of our population take these drugs. Apart from drugs, some other factors (alcohol, spoilt food etc.) can also function via a blockade of DAO as an additional risk. DAO-blockade is therefore a real epidemiological problem. Evidence is presented here for the new disease concept: Food-Induced Histaminosis.

1986

Red wine asthma: a controlled challenge study
Dahl R, Henriksen JM, Harving H.

J Allergy Clin Immunol. 1986 Dec;78(6):1126-9
Drinking red wine may provoke bronchospasm in subjects with asthma. In order to reveal some of the possible agents involved in this reaction, 18 patients with a history of red wine-induced asthma were studied. They received, in a double-blind fashion, red wine with low sulfur dioxide (SO2) and high amine, high SO2 and high amine and low SO2 and low amine content. In each challenge, the wine was administered in stepwise increasing quantities until a total of 385 ml or a fall in peak expiratory flow of greater than 15% was reached. Nine subjects demonstrated a significant fall in peak flow in one or more challenges. In all cases the most severe reaction was observed after the wine with high SO2 content. The study suggests that SO2 is the most important factor in red wine-induced asthma. It is recommended that wine labels provide information on the SO2 content.

Histamine in foods: its possible role in non-allergic adverse reactions to ingestants

Malone MH, Metcalfe DD.
N Engl Reg Allergy Proc. 1986 May-Jun; 7(3):241-5
Histamine is well recognized as a product of both mast cells and basophils. Its release from these sources in IgE-mediated reactions unquestionably contributes to the allergic response. It is often stated that ingestion of foods rich in histamine can result in absorption of sufficient histamine to provoke signs and symptoms reminiscent of an allergic reaction. A review of literature relevant to this issue suggests that certain foods do indeed contain histamine as measured by current methodology. Further, histamine ingestion in excess of 36 to 250 mg may or may not result in a clinical response which includes abdominal complaints, feelings of warmth, flushing and headache. Taken together, this evidence supports the hypothesis that ingestion of large amounts of histamine-containing foods or foods which contain the histamine precursor, histidine, under some circumstances can result in adverse reactions.

Histamine food poisoning: toxicology and clinical aspects

Taylor SL
Crit Rev Toxicol. 1986;17(2):91-128
Histamine poisoning can result from the ingestion of food containing unusually high levels of histamine. Fish are most commonly involved in incidents of histamine poisoning, although cheese has also been implicated on occasion. The historic involvement of tuna and mackerel in histamine poisoning led to the longtime usage of the term, scombroid fish poisoning, to describe this food-borne illness. Histamine poisoning is characterized by a short incubation period, a short duration, and symptoms resembling those associated with allergic reactions. The evidence supporting the role of histamine as the causative agent is compelling. The efficacy of antihistamine therapy, the allergic-like symptomology, and the finding of high levels of histamine in the implicated food suggest strongly that histamine is the causative agent. However, histamine ingested with spoiled fish appears to be much more toxic than histamine ingested in an aqueous solution. The presence of potentiators of histamine toxicity in the spoiled fish may account for this difference in toxicity. Several potentiators including other putrefactive amines such as putrescine and cadaverine have been identified. Pharmacologic potentiators may also exist; aminoguanidine and isoniazid are examples. The mechanism of action of these potentiators appears to be the inhibition of intestinal histamine-metabolizing enzymes. This enzyme inhibition causes a decrease in histamine detoxification in the intestinal mucosa and results in increased intestinal uptake and urinary excretion of unmetabolized histamine.

1985

Inhibition of human and canine diamine oxidase by drugs used in an intensive care unit: relevance for clinical side effects?

Sattler J, Hesterberg R, Lorenz W, Schmidt U, Crombach M, Stahlknecht CD.
Agents Actions. 1985 Apr;16(3-4):91-4
Three hundred and forty-one drugs, commonly used in intensive care units (ICU), were chosen for an investigation of possible activation or inhibition of the histamine metabolizing enzyme diamine oxidase (DAO). After examination of 164 substances, using both canine and human DAO in an in vitro screening test, 61 agents inhibited DAO activity to various degrees. Of these, 44 inhibited the enzyme from both species, 4 inhibited the canine enzyme only and 13 the human DAO only. No compound tested was able to enhance the enzyme activity. The inhibiting agents included representatives of all major therapeutic groups. A particularly strong inhibition was observed with the neuromuscular blocking drugs d-tubocurarine, pancuronium and alcuronium, however, the other commonly used neuromuscular blocking drug, suxamethonium, was without effect. Similarly with the cephalosporines, cefotiame and cefuroxime caused a marked inhibition of the human DAO activity, whereas another regularly-used substance of this class, cefotaxime, inhibited neither the human nor the canine enzyme in concentrations up to 10(-3) M. The observation that within a given therapeutic group some members inhibit and others do not, could be useful in choosing a therapy concept which minimizes the risk of a more severe 'histamine' reaction in seriously ill patients.

Salicylates in foods

Swain AR, Dutton SP, Truswell AS
Journal of the American Dietetic Association, 1985, 85 (8): 950–60
To determine salicylate content, 333 food items were analyzed. Foods were homogenized with 25% sodium hydroxide, allowed to stand overnight, acidified with concentrated hydrochloric acid, and then extracted with warm diethylether over 5 hours. The extract was dried and taken up in dilute sodium bicarbonate solution for analysis. Salicylic acid was separated by high performance liquid chromatography and quantified by reading at 235 nm. Salicylic acid standards were used throughout to standardize extractions and analyses. This is the most comprehensive set of data on food salicylates yet published; extraction appears to have been more complete for some foods, giving higher values than those previously published. Most fruits, especially berry fruits and dried fruits, contain salicylate. Vegetables show a wide range from 0 to 6 mg salicylate per 100 gm food (for gherkins). Some herbs and spices were found to contain very high amounts per 100 gm, e.g., curry powder, paprika, thyme, garam masala, and rosemary. Among beverages, tea provides substantial amounts of salicylate. Licorice and peppermint candies and some honeys contain salicylates. Cereals, meat, fish, and dairy products contain none or negligible amounts.

1984

Histamine liberators and the mechanisms of mediator release
Alm PE
Acta Otolaryngol Suppl. 1984; 414: 102-7

Histamine content, diamine oxidase activity and histamine methyltransferase activity in human tissues: fact or fictions?
Hesterberg R, Sattler J, Lorenz W, Stahlknecht CD, Barth H, Crombach M, Weber D
Agents Actions. 1984; 14(3-4): 325-34
To understand the role of histamine in the aetiology and pathogenesis of human diseases reliable data are urgently needed for the histamine content and for the activities of histamine-forming and -inactivating enzymes in human tissues. In order to make a substantial progress toward this aim a tissue-sampling programme during surgical interventions was carefully conceived and conducted. From March 1982 until January 1983 106 tissue specimens were taken from 56 patients who underwent surgery. Only healthy tissues, not injured or oedematous, and without adherent structures were taken by only one surgeon who was interested in this research and experienced in tissue preparation procedures in biochemistry. The times of 'warm' ischaemia during the operative procedures were visually estimated, the times between resection of the organs or specimens and deep-freezing of the tissues were precisely recorded. Compared to previous work in the literature and especially to our own work using the same assays for determination higher histamine contents were found in this study in most of the tissues, in particular in the gastrointestinal tract. Also the diamine oxidase activities were considerably higher in many organs, e.g. 3-4 times higher in the gastrointestinal tract when compared with those in publications of our group who used always the same analytical test. However, the histamine methyltransferase activities in this study were not at variance to those determined in previous investigations. Many of them were reported in this communication for the first time. Since the methods for histamine determination and those for measuring enzymic activities were not different in this study and in previous communications of our group we are convinced that the optimized tissue-sampling and -preparation techniques were responsible for the higher values in this communication. But the problem of the 'warm' ischaemia period could not be solved by sample-taking procedures of this type during operations. There are good reasons to prefer biopsy specimens for the analysis of histamine storage and metabolism in human tissues in health and disease, but - unfortunately - they are not always available.

Urinary excretion of histamine and some of its metabolites in man: influence of the diet
Keyzer JJ, Breukelman H, Wolthers BG, Heuvel M van den, Kromme N, Berg WC.
Agents Actions 1984; 15(3-4): 189–94
Urinary excretions of histamine, N tau-methylhistamine and N tau-methylimidazoleacetic acid have been determined in 10 normal subjects on 3 different diets, containing a very low protein, a low protein and a high protein amount. Foodstuffs which could contain histamine were excluded. The mean excretion of N tau-methylhistamine on the second day of each diet amounted to 0.861 mumol/24 h, 1.051 mumol/24 h and 1.378 mumol/24 h, respectively. The excretions of histamine and N tau-methylimidazoleacetic acid were not affected. In 6 normal persons on a protein low diet, the excretions of histamine, N tau-methylhistamine and N tau-methylimidazoleacetic acid have been determined for 10 days. On the fifth day, to 3 persons 200 mumol of histamine was given orally, the other 3 persons received a high protein diet. The persons receiving histamine showed a strongly enhanced excretion of N tau-methylimidazoleacetic acid, corresponding to 36.1% of the administered histamine, whereas the urinary excretions of histamine and N tau-methylhistamine were only slightly elevated. On the high protein diet, only the excretion of N tau-methylhistamine was slightly elevated. The urinary excretions of histamine in the female subjects sometimes showed unexpectedly high

values. Most probably, this phenomenon is attributable to bacterial histamine production in the urogenital tract.

1983

Agents that Release Histamine from Mast Cells
Lagunoff D, Martin TW, Read G
Annual Review of Pharmacology and Toxicology 1983, Vol. 23: 331-351

Pseudo-allergic reactions to drugs and chemicals
Schlumberger HD.
Ann Allergy. 1983 Aug; 51(2 Pt 2):317-24
Drugs can interfere with the immune system in two basically different ways: (1) they may interact with the specific recognition mechanisms of the immune system and thus induce an allergic response that is specific for the offending agent; (2) drugs may exert pharmacological effects on the immune systems which result in a response that is independent of its recognition structures or they may activate effector and amplification mechanisms that are normally triggered by specific immune processes. Allergic reactions to drugs are different from reactions that exhibit the same clinical symptoms but lack the specificity of an allergic reaction to the offending agent. It has been suggested that those non-specific reactions which mimic the signs and symptoms of allergic reactions should be classified as pseudo-allergic reactions (PAR). PAR are characterized by the following properties which differentiate them from allergic reactions. (1) The symptoms of PAR are qualitatively different from the pharmacological response of a drug and are not related to adverse reactions connected with its pharmacological and toxicological profile. (2) PAR are not specific with regard to the chemical structure of the triggering agent. (3) PAR lack transferability to other subjects of the same species. (4) In contrast to the allergic reactivity, the pseudo-allergic reactivity is not acquired but genetically predetermined. (5) Pseudo-allergic reactivity is often expressed upon the first contact with an eliciting agent. PAR are thus an expression of a pharmacological interaction of drugs or their metabolites in genetically predisposed individuals.

1980

Headache provocation by continuous intravenous infusion of histamine. Clinical results and receptor mechanisms
Krabbe AA, Olesen J.
Pain. 1980 Apr;8(2):253-9
Histamine, 0.16, 0.33 and 0.66 microgram/kg/min, was infused intravenously to 13 normal non-headache-prone volunteers, 10 patients with chronic muscle contraction headache and 25 patients with common migraine. In the normal group no patients developed pulsating headache. In the migraine group 13 patients developed severe, 9 patients moderate and 2 patients mild pulsating headache, and only 1 patient failed to develop headache at all. The muscle contraction headache patients responded intermediately. At each infusion rate the headache was of constant quality and severity as long as the infusion continued, but disappeared shortly after its termination. Injection of an H1 blocking agent, mepyramine, almost immediately abolished the headache. The H2 blocker cimetidine was much less effective, but still significantly better than placebo. The i.v. histamine infusion test is a useful model for the study of experimental vascular headache.

Blood and mast cell histamine levels in magnesium-deficient rats
Kraeuter SL, Schwartz R.
J Nutr. 1980 May; 110(5): 851-8
The number and morphology of mast cells (MCs) in the duodenal submucosa and the histamine content of blood and isolated peritoneal mast cells were estimated sequentially in male weanling Sprague-Dawley rats magnesium (Mg)-depleted for up to 48 days. Blood histamine levels increased 4--5-fold by 14 days of Mg depletion and subsequently declined to levels similar to those in pair-fed Mg-adequate controls. In the same period, the submucosal MCs continuously increased in number, beginning to plateau at 6--7 times the control number between days 36--48 of Mg deficiency. Massive MC degranulation was seen in the early stages of Mg-depletion but subsided after 16--20 days. Subsequently, the submucosal MCs appeared small and rounded. They showed reduced staining with toluidine blue indicating a deficiency in the mucopolysaccharide component of the storage granules. Histamine content of purified peritoneal MCs from Mg-deficient rats was reduced by 10 days of Mg depletion and remained at or below one-third the control level throughout the depletion period. The data suggest that the MCs remaining or developed during chronic Mg depletion are deficient in their capacity to store and secrete histamine.

1979

Respiratory distress and hypoxemia in systemic mastocytosis
Kaye WA, Passero MA
Chest. 1979; 75(1): 87-8
A 25-year-old woman with documented mastocytosis developed hypoxemia with pruritus, diarrhea, headache, and hypotension on two separate occasions. The hypoxemia appeared to be related to a massive release of histamine. Resolution of the patient's symptoms was accompanied by the return of her arterial oxygen tension to normal levels.

The role of exogenous histamine in scombroid poisoning
Motil, K. J. and Scrimshaw, N. S.
Toxicol. Lett. 1979, 3, 219
In order to investigate the role of histamine as a causative factor in scombroidpoisoning, four subjects received grapefruit juice with or without graded doses of histamine in a randomized double-blind fashion for 10 days. Eight subjects received tuna sandwiches with or without histamine in the same manner. Clinical symptoms and vital signs were recorded daily. Histaminase activity was measured in plasma eosinophils and serum.
Results demonstrated that although vital signs and histaminase activity showed no consistent pattern of change at any histamine dose, characteristic symptoms of scombroidpoisoning (severe headaches and facial flushing) were noted at the 100-, 150-, and 180-mg doses of histamine. These findings suggest that histamine is responsible for the symptoms seen in scombroidpoisoning.

In vitro inhibition of rat intestinal histamine-metabolizing enzymes
Taylor SL, Lieber ER
Food Cosmet Toxicol. 1979 Jun;17(3):237-40

1972

"Hot-dog" headache: individual susceptibility to nitrite
Henderson WR, Raskin NH
Lancet. 1972; 2 (7788): 1162-3
A patient who had noted the development of headaches shortly after eating frankfurters agreed to a series of tests aimed at determining whether the nitrites in frankfurters were the cause of his " hot-dog " headaches. He drank odourless and tasteless solutions containing 10 mg. or less of sodium nitrite or solutions identical in appearance containing 10 mg. of sodium bicarbonate. Headaches were provoked eight out of thirteen times after the ingestion of sodium nitrite, but never after the control solution. Headaches were also provoked by the ingestion of solutions containing 100 mg. of tyramine hydrochloride. The mechanism of headache production by these exogenous chemicals is uncertain.

1968

Effects of oral histamine, histidine, and diet on urinary excretion of histamine, methylhistamine, and 1-methyl-4-imidazoleacetic acid in man
Granerus, G.
Scand. J . Lab. Clin. Invest. 1968, 22 (Suppl. 104), 49

The role of tyramine in the aetiology of migraine, and related studies on the cerebral and extracerbral circulations
Hanington E, Harper AM
Headache: The Journal of Head and Face Pain, 1968, 8/3, 84–97

1967

Preliminary report on tyramine headache
Hanington
Source: British Medical Journal, May 1967, 550-551

1932

The systemic effects of histamine in man
Weiss, S., Robb, G.P., and Ellis, L.B.
Arch. Int. Med., 1932, 49, 360

THE END

Made in the USA
Monee, IL
12 August 2022